Grains
for Better Health

*Over 100 Delicious Recipes
Using Rice, Wheat, Barley,
and Other Wholesome Grains*

Maureen B. Keane

Daniella Chace

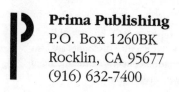

Prima Publishing
P.O. Box 1260BK
Rocklin, CA 95677
(916) 632-7400

To Goldie Caughlan, who first introduced us to whole foods. Her dedication to nutrition education has inspired a second generation of nutrition optimists.

Production by Melanie Field, Bookman Productions
Copyediting by Carol Ann Sheffield
Illustrations by Daniella Chace and Richard Sheppard
Typography by Graphic Sciences Corporation
Interior design by Paula Goldstein, Bookman Productions
Cover illustration by Dan Brown
Cover design by The Dunlavey Studio, Sacramento

Library of Congress Cataloging-in-Publication Data

Keane, Maureen.
    Grains for better health : over 100 delicious recipes using rice,
  wheat, barley, and other wholesome grains / Maureen B. Keane.
  Daniella B. Chace.
      p.   cm.
    Includes index.
    ISBN 1-55958-486-6
    1. Cookery (Cereals)   2. Grain.   I. Chace, Daniella.   II. Title.
TX808.K43   1994
641.6'31—dc20   94-6008
                                                          CIP

94   95   96   97   98   RRD   10   9   8   7   6   5   4   3   2   1
Printed in the United States of America

How to Order:

Single copies may be ordered from Prima Publishing, P.O. Box 1260BK, Rocklin, CA 95677; telephone (916) 632-7400. Quantity discounts are also available. On your letterhead, include information concerning the intended use of the books and the number of books you wish to purchase.

CONTENTS

CHAPTER 3

How to Choose a Steamer   27

CHAPTER 4

Grain Steamers   34

CHAPTER 5

In Search of the Perfect Grain   39

CHAPTER 6

Amaranth   52

CHAPTER 7

Barley   62

CHAPTER 8

Buckwheat   74

CHAPTER 9

Kamut   84

CHAPTER 10

Millet   95

CHAPTER 11

Oats   105

CHAPTER 12

Quinoa   118

CHAPTER 13

Rice   130

CHAPTER 14

Rye   156

CHAPTER 15

Spelt   166

CHAPTER 16

Teff   174

CHAPTER 17

Triticale   183

CHAPTER 18

Wheat   191

CHAPTER 19

Wild Rice   205

Acknowledgments

We would like to thank Jennifer Basye, Andi Reese Brady, Karen Blanco, and Jenn Nelson at Prima and Melanie Field at Bookman Productions for their help in publishing this book.

We would also like to thank the companies who so generously provided us with rice steamers: Aroma, Black & Decker, Hamilton Beach, Hitachi, Maverick, Panasonic, Rival, Salton, and Westbend and the friendly people at Bob's Red Mill in Oregon for their gracious assistance.

Thank you John, Micheál, and Dan, the great men who stand behind us. A special pat on the head to Maeve—your creativity with rice still amazes us.

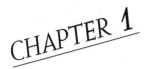

CHAPTER 1

Grains and Grain Steamers

*T*urn your rice steamer into a whole-grain steamer! Rice steamers have traditionally been used solely for white rice. In fact, if you walked into a store to purchase a rice cooker, the odds are the salesperson would tell you that they cook only white rice, not brown rice—and certainly not spelt or Kamut. Well, this simply is not true—and with a little information on the nutritional value and culinary versatility of the many fabulous whole grains available today, you will soon be on your way to making quick, healthful, and delicious meals.

Many people are not familiar with the different grains available; others may just feel they don't have the time or the know-how to cook whole grains. These unfortunate souls have been kept long enough from the enjoyment of home-cooked, fresh, whole grains! Now the grain steamer makes cooking them foolproof. By turning your rice steamer into a grain steamer, you can reap the health benefits that all whole grains have to offer. Steamers cook whole grains perfectly. No longer do you have to stand over the stove baby-sitting the cooking grain. No longer does that grain burn to the bottom of the pot or cook into a gooey mess. Every grain emerges fluffy and whole. Even the most basic steamers work well.

Expand Your Grain Vocabulary

For most of us, if it's a flour, it's wheat; if it's a flake, that means oats; and if it's a whole grain, that means rice. Some of us may have a passing familiarity with barley, but most of us have never heard of amaranth, teff, or quinoa—let alone spelt or Kamut.

Having choices when it comes to grains is important for many reasons. First, each food has its own combination of nutrients that have specific effects on the body. The wider the variety of foods in the diet, the more we increase the range of nutrients we are consuming and the better are our chances of filling all of our bodies' daily requirements. Also, many scientists believe that food allergies are developed from overuse of a single food such as wheat. Therefore, eating a variety of grains may also help in the prevention of food allergies. Some people may already know they have allergies to certain foods and must find alternatives. For example, those who have an allergy to wheat or are intolerant of gluten need wheat-free, gluten-free cereals, bread flours, and meal grains.

Last but not least, you will prevent bored taste buds. Variety in grains can make an average recipe into a gourmet meal. Botanically, there are eight thousand species of grasses that produce grains. There is a whole new world of flavors and textures to be discovered in the array of whole grains now available on the market.

Use Your Brains—Eat Grains

It's just common sense. Each type of grain has its own unique blend of fiber and nutrients. Whole grains are rich sources of

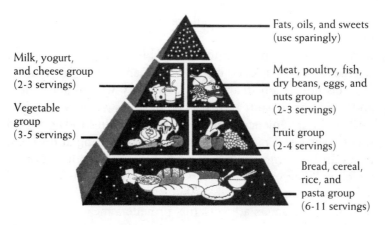

Figure 1.1   The Food Pyramid

carbohydrates, vitamins, minerals, and fiber—as well as a host of health-benefiting and cancer-fighting phytochemicals.

We have recently been told by the leading health organizations of our country as well as by medical specialists and nutritionists that we do not eat enough whole grains and that whole grains should be the major component of our daily dietary intake. Not only do we not get enough grains, they should form the base of everyone's diet. Sixty percent of our total food intake each day should be from whole grains and their products. That is what the new food pyramid from the United States Department of Agriculture is telling us (see Figure 1.1). Amazingly enough, everyone now seems to agree that this is the one step we can all take toward better health.

Modern Home Economics

Grains are great not only for our health but for our budgets too. Buying whole grains is inexpensive, literally pennies per pound, and they all but last forever, so there is very little waste. They can be purchased at your local grocery in packages, from co-ops in bulk, from health food stores, and through the mail. Most people have found that these delightful grains are fairly easy to purchase but that once they get them home and have to cook them up, things get a little more intimidating. However, an electric rice steamer or "grain steamer" can alleviate many of the problems.

Using a grain steamer is also an easy way to get variety and nutrition despite fast-paced lifestyles—a way to make healthful convenience foods. For many families today, a meal together is just a memory—now we are all eating at different times and running out the door. But starting a pot of grains, which will keep warm for hours, provides a healthful hot meal for everyone, no matter what their schedule.

Grain steamers are versatile, provide a means of cooking whole meals for those with limited cooking space or equipment, and require minimal cleanup with virtually no maintenance. Using a steamer to cook up hot meals can be a health-saving strategy for students or artists who have limited cooking facilities in dorm rooms or loft spaces.

Types of Steamers

Rice steamers appear on store shelves under a variety of names. We're going to refer to rice steamers, food steamers, rice cookers, and vegetables steamers as "grain steamers" from here on out.

We have found that there are just two main types of machines, with minor variations within each category: metal rice cookers and plastic rice steamers. The metal units are similar to Crock-Pots and often come with a perforated insert which gives them the ability to be used as steamers. The plastic units cook by steaming alone. They do a wonderful job of making fluffy, moist, whole grains. Chapter 3 tells you how to select a steamer if you don't already own one.

Whole Grains for Health

Grains, or cereals, are members of the grass family. The grains are actually many small, separate, dry fruits. Wheat, barley, oats, and rye have always been important grains in the Middle East and Europe, while rice has long been the staple grain of Asia. Maize, or corn, has been a staple of the Americas, and sorghum and millet the main grains of Africa. Quinoa, amaranth, wild rice, and buckwheat are sometimes called "pseudocereals" because their culinary uses and nutritional benefits are much like those of the cereal grains. However, they come from different botanical families.

All grains have the same basic structure. The outer seed coat comprises several thin layers that make up the epidermis. Then comes the aleurone layer, which contains the oil, minerals, protein, and vitamins. Under that is the endosperm, the organ that stores most of the carbohydrates and protein. This forms the bulk of the grain and is the "starchy" part of the kernel. Each kernel also contains a small, fibrous germ layer, called the scutellum. This is the part of the grain which allows it to sprout and grow into a plant.

Whole grains are valued for their carbohydrate, protein, healthful fat (oil), vitamin, mineral, and fiber content. A refined grain does not have all the nutrients the whole grain has; therefore, minimal processing is desirable, nutritionally speaking.

Processing—Less Means More

Grains have been milled for thousands of years. In earliest times, people used rocks to crush the tough layers of the grain. Later, water-powered mills did the job; and eventually, electric milling processes were used. Milling can cause a loss of nutritional value due to the hulling and degermination processes. The form into which a grain is processed also has an effect on its nutritional value. Some grains may be refined in such a way that they have lost their most healthful components. Highly refined grains have had their bran and germ removed.

Grains can be steel cut, rolled, flaked, presteamed, and ground into meals and flours. The indigestible hulls are the first part to go in processing. Removing this husk makes them easier to cook and chew. Removing the hulls, cutting, and rolling have minimal effect on the nutrients.

The next layer of grain to be lost is the bran. The bran has many health benefits since it is made of soluble and insoluble fiber, which assists in bowel cleansing, cholesterol regulation, and digestion.

The germ is the other nutritious component that can be lost in the processing of grains. The germ contains healthful oils, a majority of the grain's vitamin content, valuable minerals, and known and unknown phytochemicals. We are just now discovering the importance of phytochemicals, healthful nutrients that appear to be preserved in whole grains during the steaming process.

Grains can be eaten at almost every stage of the milling process, given enough cooking. Yet most of the grain products on the market today are highly refined to the point of serious nutrient depletion. Some refined grains have been enriched, fortified, or have had fiber added back into them. But when you see the word "enriched" on a food label, this should be a red flag in your mind that this is *not* a whole grain product and not nearly as nutritious as its original form. To sum it up, the whole grain is always going to be a more healthful choice than its refined counterpart. And because whole grains are such an important part of our diet, it is imperative that we understand which grains are of the highest nutritional quality.

In a Nutshell

The purpose of this book is to introduce you to some of the more unusual grains, to provide you with delicious, quick, and simple recipes for incorporating them into your daily diet, and to put you in touch with mail order sources for some hard-to-find grains. Each grain chapter contains a bit of folklore, history, and scientific fact, along with practical health information such as the vitamin and mineral content. In highlighting the specific food components and their benefits, from fiber to phytochemicals, we hope to illustrate the relationship of these foods to the prevention and healing of disease.

Each chapter also teaches you how to purchase, properly wash, and store grains. For each grain you will find basic cooking instructions, a breakfast cereal, a pilaf recipe, a cold salad recipe, and a selection of our favorite dishes. Health was our number-one priority in developing these recipes. However, we feel that they are also superior in flavor and texture. In line with the new food pyramid, they are based on carbohydrate-rich grains, with special attention to keeping the fat, sodium, and sugar levels low. They are easy to put together, even with minimal kitchen equipment or cooking experience. With about the same amount of effort and money you would use to go out for fast food, you will be making healthful, hot, home-made dishes.

Nutrition Facts

For those of you who are interested in going further with calculations of your dietary intake, it is important to understand the food label information provided. Each recipe has been analyzed for its nutritional content. This is presented in the new FDA food label format for quick reference. It includes such helpful information as the number of calories that come from fat. For example, let's say we have a quarter cup of wheat germ, which contains 108 calories. Wheat germ contains 3 grams of fat, and we know that each gram of fat contributes 9 calories. So there are 3×9 or 27 calories from fat—as would be shown in the food label. To calculate the *percentage* of calories from fat, we divide the fat calories by total calories or 27 fat calories / 108 total calories = .25 or 25%. This means that 25% of the calories in wheat germ come from fat. The remaining 75% come from other components such as protein, starches, and sugars.

The label also tells us how much protein each serving contains as well as the levels of vitamins A and C, calcium, and iron. The fat, cholesterol, and sodium percentages are based on 2,000 daily calorie intakes. For carbohydrates and fiber, the percentage reflects the minimum amount you should eat each day. The % Daily Value amounts are evaluations of how much each nutrient in one serving contributes to the total amount of that nutrient recommended for each day. In other words, 300 milligrams (mg) of sodium accounts for 13% of the 2,400 mg (or less) recommended daily allowance.

Fat in the diet has been getting a lot of press lately and for good reason. But please keep in mind that the amount of fat in each meal is only part of your dietary intake, and it is OK to go under or above your target now and then as long as you are aiming for a 30%-or-less fat ratio for your total daily caloric intake.

We did not include salt in most of the recipes. One teaspoon of salt contains 2,000 mg of sodium. To calculate how much sodium you have added to your recipe, multiply the number of teaspoons of salt by 2,000 and divide by the number of servings.

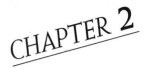

Health and Grains

*I*f our bodies are likened to machines then food is the fuel that powers the engine. When the fuel is of poor quality, the engine sputters and backfires, and the machine does not run or performs poorly. When the fuel is too rich, the engine becomes sluggish and clogged. Either way, the machine becomes prone to breakdowns and never operates at peak efficiency. If your personal machine needs tune-ups too often or if it doesn't accelerate like it used to, don't blame worn out engine parts; it may be the fuel you are using.

Whole grains are some of the best fuels you can put into your engine's tank. Not only are they excellent sources of time-release energy, they also contain the B vitamins necessary to utilize that energy. Grains are also excellent sources of fiber, which prevents clogs and keeps things flowing cleanly through the pipes of the system.

But in real life, food is more than a fuel that provides energy and growth factors. It is a complex mixture of compounds that also protect the body from the often hostile environment of the modern world. These compounds are called phytochemicals, and most of them are still largely unknown or unrecognized. They cannot be duplicated in the laboratory or obtained from a pill. They can be obtained only through food.

In this chapter we are going to explore the nutritional qualities of grains. We will look at their nutrient contents, including vitamins, minerals, carbohydrates, proteins, fiber, and phytochemicals, and see how these nutrients prevent disease and how they can be used to treat disease.

Carbohydrates

When a plant absorbs energy from the sun, that energy is stored in the chemical bonds of molecules called carbohydrates. Carbohydrates are essential nutrients that are chiefly obtained from plant foods. They are a source of energy and the major source of fiber in the human diet. There are three general types of carbohydrates: simple carbohydrates, digestible complex carbohydrates, and indigestible carbohydrates.

Simple Carbohydrates

Sugar molecules, or simple carbohydrates, are the building blocks of complex carbohydrates. When the body digests food for energy, it breaks down the complex carbohydrates into their component sugars. All complex carbohydrates must be reduced to simple sugars before they can be absorbed by the digestive tract.

Glucose is a simple sugar that is one of the main fuels of the body and the only form of carbohydrate that can be transported by the blood to the tissues. For example, the skeletal muscle, heart muscle, digestive system, and all other systems are powered by glucose. The central nervous system uses about nine tablespoons of glucose each day and the red blood cells need about three tablespoons.

When glucose enters the bloodstream, the pancreas releases a hormone called insulin. Insulin allows glucose to pass through cell membranes to where the glucose is "burned" for energy. Without insulin, cells could float in glucose but still starve to death.

Digestible Complex Carbohydrates

Digestible complex carbohydrates, sometimes called starches or polysaccharides, are made up of chains of glucose. When these chains reach the human digestive tract, enzymes secreted by the digestive system are able to reduce the complex carbohydrates to simple carbohydrates. A good example of this occurs when you chew a piece of bread. At first the bread is only slightly sweet. But the longer you chew, the sweeter the bread becomes. This is because the complex carbohydrates of the bread are being broken down into sugars by the digestive enzymes of the saliva. These sugars are then absorbed into the bloodstream and carried into individual cells, where the chemical bonds are broken and the stored energy released.

Complex carbohydrates are a time-release form of energy. The glucose made from them enters the bloodstream slowly. This results in insulin also being released slowly, an important plus for those with diabetes or hypoglycemia.

Indigestible Complex Carbohydrates

Some types of complex carbohydrates resist breakdown by the enzymes secreted by the human digestive tract. They are therefore called indigestible complex carbohydrates. This type of carbohydrate enters the colon or large intestine in much the same form in which it was eaten. Indigestible complex carbohydrates form most of the fiber in the human diet.

Cellulose, a type of indigestible carbohydrate, is the most abundant carbohydrate found on earth. It forms the framework of plants. Other important indigestible carbohydrates include beta glucans, gums, and pectin.

Fiber

Dietary fiber is not a substance that can be defined like a chemical. It comprises a diverse group of plant substances that vary greatly in composition from one species to another and even from one plant to another within a species. In general, dietary fiber is a generic term that describes a group of carbohydrates or compounds derived from carbohydrates that show three properties: they resist digestion by human digestive enzymes, they are able to reach the colon, and they have some effect on gastrointestinal function. Almost all fiber found in the human diet comes from the cell walls of cereals and other seeds, fruits, and vegetables. Each plant has its own unique blend of fiber.

Dietary fiber can be divided into two main subclasses. They are commonly called soluble fiber and insoluble fiber.

Soluble Fiber

Soluble fiber is a group of fibers that are able to dissolve in the watery contents of the gastrointestinal tract. They form gels (are viscous) and are easily fermented by the bacteria that live in the colon. This type of fiber is able to exert its effects on the entire body.

Soluble fiber is broken down by the colonic bacteria to produce carbohydrates that are then fermented to produce gases (carbon dioxide, hydrogen, and methane), lactic acid, and short chain fatty acids (SCFAs—mainly acetate, propionate, and butyrate). These fermentation products can then interact with the cells of the colon or be absorbed into the bloodstream. In particular, SCFAs can travel to the liver, where they can reduce cholesterol production and influence the metabolism of glucose and fats. Diets rich in soluble fiber are associated with lower serum cholesterol, decreased insulin levels in the blood, and increased feeling of fullness after eating.

Barley and oats are two of the best grain sources of soluble fiber.

Insoluble Fiber

Insoluble fiber is a group of fibers that do not dissolve in the watery contents of the gastrointestinal tract. They are nonviscous and resist fermentation by the bacteria of the colon. Insoluble fiber affects the gastrointestinal tract only locally. It increases the mass of the feces, increases the frequency of bowel movements, and reduces the amount of time it takes for food to travel through the digestive system. Diets rich in insoluble fiber are associated with a reduced risk of colon and rectal cancer, decreased constipation, and reduced blood pressure.

Whole wheat, brown rice, and amaranth are excellent sources of insoluble fiber.

Protein

Protein is the substance out of which body tissue is made. Proteins are very large and complex molecules that are made up of building blocks called amino acids. There are only twenty-two different amino acids. The human body's estimated ten to fifty thousand different proteins are all made up from different combinations of the same twenty-two amino acids.

There are ten essential amino acids. They are called essential because they cannot be made by the body but must be obtained from the diet. If the body is deprived of even one of the essential amino acids, it cannot synthesize protein.

In the United States, however, the problem we face is not a lack of protein in the diet but an excess. We eat too much animal protein, which comes attached to too much animal fat. This fat may be responsible for many of the chronic diseases that afflict people in the developed world. We need to increase our high-carbohydrate sources of protein and decrease greatly our high-fat sources of protein.

Protein and Grains

Grains, along with legumes, are excellent lowfat, high-carbo-hydrate sources of protein. Grains contain all of the ten essential amino acids. However, grains do not contain the same amounts of amino acids as found in animal flesh and products. For example, grains contain lower amounts of lysine and threonine. Since these two amino acids are found in higher amounts in legumes and seeds as well as in milk and eggs, the missing amounts can be easily supplied in the diet. Only diets that are dangerously low in calories are likely to be deficient in protein.

Grains and Fats

Plants store energy as carbohydrates; animals store energy as fats. Fats are concentrated forms of energy: each gram of fat provides 9 kilocalories while each gram of carbohydrate provides only 4 grams per kilocalorie.

Grains, however, are the seeds of cereal plants and they must contain enough food energy for a developing plant. This food energy must necessarily be concentrated and is therefore present in the form of fats. Grain usually is composed of 1 to 3% fats. Amaranth has the least at 0.5%, followed by wild rice at 0.7%, barley at 1%, rye at 1.7%, rice at 1.9%, wheat at 2%, buckwheat at 2.4%, and millet at 2.9%. On average, half of the oil found in seeds is composed of linoleic acid. Linoleic acid is an essential fatty acid that the human body cannot manufacture on its own.

Grains are very poor sources of saturated fats. What is important about grains, however, is not the kinds of fats that they contain but how the compounds found in grains affect fat absorption and cholesterol production in the body. For example, sitosterol is a phytochemical found in rice that competes for absorption with cholesterol.

Grains and Vitamins

Vitamins are substances that are needed in very small amounts but that cannot always be manufactured by the body and so must come from food. Unlike people, plants *can* manufacture vitamins, from the nutrients provided by the soil.

Whole grains are not only excellent sources of energy in the form of complex carbohydrates but good sources of the B-complex vitamins, which are necessary for the body to release that energy. Many grains are also good sources of the antioxidant vitamin E.

Grains and Minerals

Grains are good sources of many minerals, including calcium, magnesium, copper, zinc, and iron. However, grains are also good sources of phytic acid, a compound that binds some of the minerals and makes them unavailable for absorption. Vitamin C makes more of these minerals available. In order to get the most nutritive value out of grains, be sure to include a source of vitamin C with your meal. Sources of vitamin C can be found in chapter 5.

Phytochemicals

One of the most exciting features of grains is the recent discovery of phytochemicals (phyto = plant) in them. These substances are not minerals or vitamins; they are naturally occurring compounds found in grains and other plants that the human body has learned to use in various ways. These compounds are not related chemically to each other. Each one has unique properties that researchers have only begun to discover. They have been called nutraceuticals and anutrients as well as phytochemicals.

Phytochemicals found in grains include phytoestrogens, which can reduce the effects of menopause and reduce the incidence of breast cancer; phytic acid, which may reduce cancer risk; and saponins, which may reduce elevated cholesterol levels.

Health and Grains

Arthritis, Inflammatory

Inflammatory types of arthritis may be triggered or aggravated by certain foods. Wheat is one of the main culprits. By substituting oatmeal, buckwheat, rice, and other grains, you can still achieve a high-fiber diet while avoiding wheat. Some individuals who are sensitive to wheat can tolerate spelt and Kamut, which are in the wheat family. Rice bran is an excellent substitute for wheat bran.

Birth Defects

Neural tube defects, including spina bifida and anencephaly, may be avoided by eating just 0.4 mg of folate each day. This nutrient must be included in the diet of women who are of child-bearing age because by the time a woman realizes she is pregnant, it is too late in gestation to prevent the birth defects. Grains that are good sources of folate include wheat germ, amaranth, and triticale.

Cancer Prevention

Numerous government agencies and health organizations recommend that Americans increase their consumption of fiber-rich foods. High-fiber foods such as whole grains appear to prevent colorectal cancer and are implicated in the prevention of breast, pancreatic, and prostate cancer.

When the soluble, fermentable fiber found in some grains reaches the colon, it is broken down by the bacteria that reside there, producing metabolites such as the previously mentioned fatty acids acetate, butyrate, and propionate. These compounds decrease the pH of the colon, which protects the colon from damage by bile acids.

Oats, rice, and wheat germ appear to increase the detoxification and excretion of the female hormone estrogen. Estrogen in some way promotes the development of breast cancer.

Buckwheat contains a flavone called rutin. Flavonoids have been found to inhibit the formation of cancer.

Celiac Disease

Celiac disease is an inherited inability to tolerate gliadin and prolamine, two amino acids found chiefly in the gluten portion of wheat, oats, barley, and rye. The grain of choice for celiacs is rice. If you suffer from celiac disease, substitute brown rice for other grains and rice bran for wheat bran.

Some grains, such as amaranth, teff, and quinoa, are promoted as "essentially gluten free." For the person who is gluten intolerant, this is not good enough. Since even minute amounts of gluten can damage the colon of celiacs and may promote gastrointestinal cancers, it is best to pass on all grains except rice.

The grain steamer makes it possible to cook perfect rice in many different ways. Rice farina can be substituted for hot wheat cereals or oatmeal. Rice bran is a better source of insoluble fiber than wheat bran. Rice flour can replace wheat flours in steamed puddings. The chapter on rice includes a list of ingredients to avoid if you suffer from celiac disease.

Constipation

Constipation usually responds to a change in diet. The traditional advice is to add a heaping tablespoon of bran to your diet each day. Although wheat bran is usually recommended, rice bran may actually be superior. When adding bran, start with half a tablespoon and gradually increase. Also drink 8 to 10 glasses of water each day.

Rice and wheat bran are rich in insoluble fiber. It is thought that the fiber acts by increasing the mass of the feces, making it easier for the colon to move, and by stimulating the wall of the colon. Oat bran, which is rich in insoluble fiber, also has laxative properties although not as much.

Constipation aggravates diverticular disease and hemorrhoids. By increasing the fiber in your diet, you also decrease the chance of suffering from these ills.

Diabetes

A high-fiber diet can help to regulate blood insulin levels in diabetics, thereby preventing the development of side effects. Diets rich in soluble fiber are especially recommended. Grains that are rich in soluble fiber are barley and oats.

Whole grains are also good sources of chromium, a mineral that the body needs to regulate glucose. Niacin, thiamin, and pyridoxine, also found in whole grains, are important to sugar metabolism.

Hypoglycemia

Whole grains and other high-fiber, starchy foods delay gastric emptying, which reduces the rate at which glucose is absorbed—regulating blood glucose levels and preventing the dips that cause hypoglycemia. This appears to be the result of the soluble fiber present in whole grains. Grains highest in soluble fiber include oats, rice, and barley.

High Blood Cholesterol (Heart Disease)

Oats, brown rice, and barley are associated with the ability to lower blood cholesterol levels. Much of this is due to the soluble fiber present in these grains. However, other compounds found in these grains also aid in lowering blood cholesterol levels.

- The bran in brown rice and unpearled barley contains *tocotrienol,* a form of vitamin E that may be able to prevent the liver from producing too much cholesterol.
- Rice bran also contains *cycloartenol, beta sitosterol,* and *oryzanol,* compounds which reduce cholesterol production.
- Oat bran contains beta glucans, which are believed to be partially responsible for that food's famous cholesterol-lowering properties.
- Oats and quinoa contain saponins which, in addition to antibiotic activity, also may lower cholesterol.
- Amaranth, which is highest in insoluble fiber, contains a compound called squalene, which is thought to reduce serum cholesterol by inhibiting HMG CoA reductase, an enzyme which regulates cholesterol production.
- Barley, oats, and wheat are high in the amino acid arginine. Arginine may help to reduce blood cholesterol.

High Blood Pressure (Hypertension)

Some, but not all, hypertensives are sensitive to salt. Each teaspoon of salt contains 2,000 mg of sodium, which is ten times the amount of sodium the average person needs each day. Unless salt is added, all grains are naturally low in sodium.

Magnesium is often used to treat elevated blood pressure. Whole grains are one of the best sources of magnesium. Fiber is another food component that may decrease blood pressure.

Infertility

Oats are rich in the amino acid arginine and the mineral zinc. Other grains are rich in vitamin C and pyridoxine. These nutrients can reduce nonspecific sperm agglutination, improve sperm motility, and significantly increase sperm count.

Irritable Bowel Syndrome (IBS)

A high-insoluble-fiber diet can help to reduce the symptoms of both diarrhea and constipation. The fiber acts to normalize the gut. In one study, 3 tablespoons of wheat bran reduced symptoms in patients.

One of the major causes of IBS may be food allergy or intolerance. The most common triggers include dairy products, wheat, corn, coffee, tea, chocolate, potatoes, onions, and citrus fruits. If wheat is a trigger, you may want to eliminate rye and triticale as well. Brown rice, rice polish, and rice bran will supply the fiber you need without irritating the gut.

Kidney Stones

A high-fiber diet has been associated with a decrease in stone formation. In one study, Japanese researchers found that as little as ⅓ ounce of rice bran twice a day eaten for an average of five years decreased kidney stone reoccurrence sixfold.

Menopausal Symptoms

Wheat germ is rich in compounds called phytoestrogens. These compounds mimic estrogens, relieving the symptoms of menopause without having the cancer-promoting effects of actual estrogen.

Menstrual Problems

According to Dr. Judith Wurtman, research scientist at M.I.T., eating carbohydrates has been shown to reduce the symptoms of pre-menstrual syndrome (PMS). To prevent heavy flow, add manganese-rich foods. Cereals are rich in manganese.

Stress

Both mental and physical stress increase the need for certain nutrients which can be found in grains. These include choline, which is needed to form acetylcholine, a neurotransmitter;

tryptophan, an amino acid needed to form serotonin, another neurotransmitter in the brain; zinc and B-6, which may be lost in the urine during stress; pantothenic acid, which is needed by the adrenal gland under stress; iron, which can be lost by chelation of acids which are then lost in the urine; magnesium, which is reduced by elevated free fatty acid levels in the blood due to stress; and potassium, which is needed for stress hormone production.

Rice appears to contain small amounts of a natural form of Valium, although it is not known if it can affect the body.

Ulcers

Societies which consume high-fiber diets have the least incidence of ulcers. Researchers have found that unpolished rice reduced the amount of acid in the stomach. There is also evidence that a high-fiber diet actually helps to heal ulcers and prevent relapses.

Weight Reduction and Maintenance

Researchers think that fiber reduces the amount of food eaten by a number of ways. Fiber fills the stomach, giving a feeling of fullness, and triggers the release of peptides that regulate appetite, including cholecystokinin and pancreatic polypeptide. Fermentation by-products formed from the fiber or some as yet unidentified compound bound to the fiber may also be responsible for the appetite-blunting effects.

Weight Gain

The starches in grains are a time-release form of sugar, which supplies calories without fat for the individual who wishes to gain weight. The proteins in grains are also fat-free and therefore much heart healthier for those who wish to increase muscle weight.

Prescription for Health

We have seen how various components of grains can have effects on a number of disease states. Does this mean that you should treat grains as a medicine instead of a food? Yes and no. The electric grain steamer will definitely not replace your doctor. However, if you use your steamer on a regular basis, you may be seeing your doctor a lot less.

Remember, all whole foods nourish the body in ways other than providing just calories for energy and vitamins and minerals for growth. All foods have other compounds that can exert beneficial effects. The phytochemicals mentioned in this chapter are just a small sample of those presently identified. Researchers have barely scratched the surface when it comes to understanding all of the health implications of plant foods. But you do not have to understand the chemistry to enjoy the benefits. Just expand your grain vocabulary and let your body reap the rewards.

Grain Sources of Vitamins

Thiamin

Thiamin, or vitamin B-1, is a member of the B-complex family. Thiamin is sometimes called the anti-neuritic vitamin because it is necessary for the normal functioning of the nervous system. It is also needed for the body to release energy from food, so individuals who use more energy and eat more calories need more thiamin.

Best grain sources of thiamin: wheat germ, triticale, rice bran and polish, Kamut, spelt, teff, millet, oats, rye, and brown rice.

Riboflavin

Riboflavin, or vitamin B-2, is also a member of the B-complex family. Like thiamin and niacin, it is water soluble and involved in the production of energy from food.

Best grain sources of riboflavin: wheat germ, quinoa, rye, millet, and amaranth.

Niacin

Niacin, or vitamin B-3, is another B-complex vitamin. Like riboflavin and thiamin, niacin is needed for energy production. **Best grain sources of niacin:** wheat germ, brown rice, hulled barley, millet, rye, wheat, rice polish and bran, Kamut, spelt, and buckwheat.

Pyridoxine

Pyridoxine, or vitamin B-6, is a B-complex vitamin that helps the body use protein to build body tissue and that aids in the metabolism of fat. Women frequently consume less than 70% of the recommended daily allowance (RDA). **Best grain sources of pyridoxine:** wheat germ, rice polish, brown rice, rye, amaranth, and wild rice.

Folate

Folate, or folic acid, is one of the B vitamins. It is essential for the manufacture of red and white blood cells in the bone marrow and helps in the formation of genetic material within body cells. Folate will also aid in the prevention of neural tube defects in children when taken by their mothers before conception. **Best grain sources of folate:** wheat germ, amaranth, triticale, rye, millet, and wild rice.

Vitamin E

Vitamin E is a fat-soluble vitamin that is now gaining attention as an antioxidant. One study has shown that 45% of affluent elderly people consumed less than 75% of the RDA. **Best grain sources of vitamin E:** amaranth, wheat germ, whole wheat, oats, and rye.

Ascorbic Acid

Ascorbic acid, or vitamin C, is a water-soluble vitamin that is necessary for the formation of collagen, the protein that forms bones, cartilage, muscle, and blood vessels. It is involved in the maintenance of capillaries, bones, and teeth, and because it is a strong antioxidant, it protects the tissues of the body from free radical damage. When added to a meal, vitamin C increases the absorption of iron and other minerals from cereal and vegetable sources. **Best grain source of ascorbic acid:** amaranth.

Pantothenic Acid

Pantothenic acid belongs to the B-complex family. It is part of Coenzyme A, an enzyme that is necessary for the release of energy from carbohydrates and fatty acids. It is involved in the synthesis of cholesterol and of some hormones. **Best grain sources of pantothenic acid:** wheat germ and triticale.

Grain Sources of Minerals

Calcium

In addition to having its well-known function of building bones and teeth, calcium also is needed for the blood-clotting process, is involved in the transport function of cell membranes and the release of neurotransmitters at the synaptic junctions of nerves, and is required for nerve transmission and for regulation of the heartbeat. **Best grain source of calcium:** teff.

Magnesium

Magnesium is necessary for the production and transfer of energy for protein synthesis. It also is involved in nerve transmission and muscle contraction and is a cofactor in numerous enzyme systems.

Best grain sources of magnesium: wheat germ, buckwheat, millet, quinoa, brown rice, rye, triticale, and amaranth.

Iron

Iron carries oxygen out of the lungs to the body tissues and carries carbon dioxide away from the cells to the lungs. Iron is also necessary for cellular respiration and for proper functioning of the immune system.
Best grain sources of iron: wheat germ, quinoa, amaranth, and triticale.

Chromium

Chromium is an essential trace mineral necessary for normal carbohydrate metabolism. It is involved in the regulation of blood glucose levels and is closely associated with the hormone insulin. It has been estimated that Americans eat only half of the recommended chromium intake. The amount of chromium in foods decreases with processing.
Best grain source of chromium: barley.

Copper

Copper is a part of many enzymes. It is involved in the development and maintenance of the skeleton and cardiovascular system, the central nervous system and its function, blood cell function, and hair growth and pigmentation.
Best grain sources of chromium: barley, teff, quinoa, buckwheat, millet, and triticale.

Zinc

Marginal deficiency may be widespread in the United States. Zinc is involved with over seventy enzymes. Zinc is important in the manufacture of protein and assists in wound healing, blood formation, and general growth and maintenance of all tissues. Zinc also participates in the metabolism of nucleic acids and the synthesis of proteins as well as cell membranes. **Best grain sources of zinc**: wheat germ, triticale, rye, millet, and wild rice.

Silicon

Silicon is very important in bone formation. Animals with a silicon deficiency have a bone matrix that is transparent and less calcified. Whole grain cereals are one of the best sources of silicon.

Selenium

Selenium is an important part of the enzyme glutathione peroxidase. This enzyme protects the blood cells from oxygen damage. As an antioxidant, it works with vitamin E to protect the cell and its organelles from free radical damage. The amount of selenium in foods is directly proportional to the amount of selenium in the soil it in which they grew. Whole grains are the major source of selenium in the American diet.

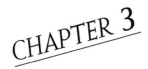

CHAPTER 3

How to Choose
a Steamer

*I*n the past few years, a multitude of steaming machines have appeared on the market. When viewed from outside of the carton, all of these machines looks very similar. It is easy to pick up the cheapest or the largest and assume you have got the best deal. Unfortunately, people often find out which features they want or need the hard way: after they have bought a machine. This chapter will help you to evaluate your needs before buying.

Types of Steamers

Remember, the manufacturers may call these machines rice cookers, rice steamers, food steamers, or vegetable steamers. But for the sake of simplicity we are referring to all of them as grain steamers.

The good news is that all of the grain steamers we tested worked very well. They all produced fluffy, separate grains of

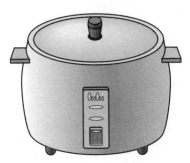

Figure 3.1 Metal steamer

brown rice with a minimum of fuss. However, some were better than others in cooking other whole grains or in cooking
smaller amounts of grains. Since steamers are relatively inexpensive, you may want to purchase two if your needs vary.

All steamers work on the same basic principle. A remov-
able rice bowl sits on top of a heat source. The metal heating
element senses when the liquid has steamed away and automatically shuts off. The amount of water added to the machine
acts much like a timer. More water is added to grains that require more cooking time, such as hulled barley, wild rice, or
oat groats. Quick-cooking grains, such as bulgur, couscous, or
scotch-cut oats, require less water.

There are basically two types of steamers available today:
round-shaped steamers with metal rice bowls and plastic
steamers with plastic rice bowls.

Metal Steamers

The metal steamer is probably the type of grain steamer most
people are familiar with. It is round and often has a white exterior. Hitachi, Aroma, and Salton make steamers of this type in
a variety of sizes. The lid is made of metal or glass, and a re-
movable metal rice bowl sits on top of a heating element. This
element heats the contents of the rice bowl and "senses" the
amount of water in the bowl. When the water has boiled away,

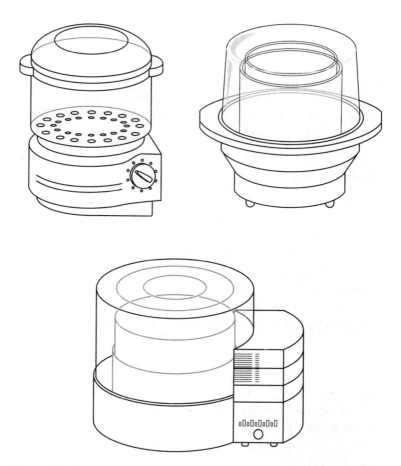

Figure 3.2 Plastic steamers

the machine automatically switches to warm. This warm cycle gently steams the grains and finishes the cooking process. Grains can be left for a number of hours on the warm cycle.

The amount of water added to the rice bowl determines the length of the cooking time. Longer-cooking grains will need more water added initially. The amount of water this type of machine uses is similar to the amount of water needed by pan cooking methods. This machine allows you to add the recommended amount of liquid and grain to the rice bowl, cover, turn on the machine, and forget about it.

Almost all of the machines come with a steaming tray that will allow you to steam vegetables. Not all machines come with an on/off switch. Some of these grain steamers are multi-purpose machines. They steam vegetables, cook rice, slow cook, and even stir fry.

Plastic Steamers

Plastic steamers come in two shapes: oval and round. With this type, a plastic rice bowl sits on top of a water reservoir which is heated by a metal element. Water poured into the reservoir produces the steam which heats the contents of the rice bowl. The raw grain and cooking liquid are added to the rice bowl. When the reservoir steams dry, the machine turns off. Since the steam is generated by a separate pool of water, only the amount of liquid needed to be absorbed by the grain is added to the bowl. A good rule of thumb is 1 part liquid to 1 part raw grain. Grains that double their size during cooking need double the water; grains that triple their volume need triple the water.

Some machines have only one water reservoir. Water that steams off during cooking condenses and re-enters the reservoir where it is used again, thereby increasing the maximum time the machine can steam. Other machines have two reservoirs: an inner reservoir which is filled at the start and an outer which gathers the "used" water. Since the water cannot be recycled, this type of machine has a shorter steaming time. With some grains it may be necessary to refill the reservoir and restart the machine.

A handy feature of many of these steamers is a timer. Machines with a timer will usually cook for up to 60 or 70 minutes. The machine turns off when the timer runs down or the reservoir steams dry.

The plastic rice bowl is very easy to clean. Since the heat is supplied only by the hot steam, grains never stick to the bottom of the bowl. Some spices can, however, stain the plastic bowl.

All of these machines come with a plastic vegetable steaming tray.

Points to Remember When Buying a Steamer

How you plan to use your steamer will help you determine the best machine for you. Is the automatic turn-off function appealing? You should consider a machine with a timer. If you plan on using your machine as a double boiler, choose a plastic machine with only one reservoir. They are designed so that it is easier to add water to prolong cooking time.

Some steamers do much more than just cook grains. One model was a rice steamer, vegetable steamer, slow cooker, and stir fryer. Another was a bread machine that cooked rice. However, it is difficult to perform all these very different tasks well with only one temperature setting. Pick the function you need most and buy for that. Machines that promise to do everything usually do nothing well.

Guidelines for Choosing a Steamer

1. *How many cups of grain will the rice bowl hold?* If you regularly cook six or more cups of whole grain at once, consider a metal machine with a capacity of ten or more cups. A large-capacity metal steamer will allow the amount of water necessary to cook whole grains without splattering water all over the counter. It will cook the grain, turn itself off, and hold the grain on warm until you are ready to serve it.

   If you cook only a few cups at a time, consider a plastic machine. Grain will not stick to the bottom of the bowl so no grain is lost in cooking. If you steam grains for one, a plastic steamer is a must. The size of the machine on the outside can sometimes be deceiving, so be sure to read the booklet that comes with the steamer to determine its cooking capacity.

2. *How sturdy is the machine?* Is the rice bowl made of good quality material? Is it sturdy and scratch resistant or thin, brittle, and easily marked? Do all the parts fit together easily and tightly? Loose fitting lids mean loss of steam, decreased cooking time, and with metal machines, a mess on the countertop.

3. *What is the shape of the rice bowl?* Is it oval or round? Deep or shallow? Steamers with oval bowls take up more counter space than round steamers but will accommodate longer pieces of vegetables, chicken, or fish. It is easier to stir grains with a shallow bowl; but if you steam only a cup of grain, a deeper bowl with the same capacity will give better results.

4. *How large is the machine?* Will it take up a lot of counter space? How easily can it be stored?

5. *If plastic, does the machine have one or two reservoirs?* Models with two reservoirs will steam for only 35 minutes, and then more water must be added. While this time is adequate for steaming vegetables, it is not enough for most whole grains. Choose a machine with only one water reservoir.

6. *Does the machine have a drip pan?* A drip pan is used with the vegetable steamer tray of plastic machines. It prevents food particles from sticking to the heating element. The second reservoir on some machines prevents food particles from the vegetable steaming tray from reaching the heating element. In machines with only one reservoir, a plastic drip pan serves the same function. It is placed under the vegetable tray and collects used water and food particles.

7. *What is the maximum steaming time?* Longer-cooking grains require additional water. Some machines are not large enough to hold all the water needed for extra cooking time. Plastic machines with two reservoirs steam for an average of 30 minutes. In order to cook some whole grains,

it is necessary to refill and restart the machine. Machines with timers run the longest, 60 to 70 minutes. If the water in the reservoir runs out before the timer goes off, the machine automatically turns off so that nothing burns.

8. *How childproof is the machine?* If you have young children, a machine with a coiled cord that does not dangle near curious hands can prevent serious burns. Some models also have a cool exterior shell that may be safer for those with children.

9. *What kind of grain will your family cook in the steamer?* Metal steamers cook brown rice and groats best. Plastic machines are great not only for whole groats but also quick-cooking grains such as buckwheat, scotch oats, bulgur, rolled cereals, and delicate small grains such as amaranth and teff.

10. *Does the machine have an on/off switch?* Although a button to turn the machine on seems a basic necessity, many machines do not have one. To turn on the machine, you plug it in. If your kitchen layout makes it difficult to reach the electrical outlet, you may be better off with a machine that has an on/off switch. However, a machine without a switch can be connected to an extension cord with an on/off switch.

Remember, look before you buy. Go to the store and examine a few models before you make your choice. We have found that price does not always determine how many features you get. However, one of our favorite machines does not even have an on/off switch. It just "feels" right and gets the job done with a minimum of fuss. Can't argue with that.

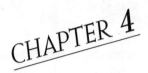

CHAPTER 4

Grain Steamers

Food steamers have been around for many years in one form or another but are just starting to be discovered by the general public. These handy machines fit right into the kitchen of the 90s because they are economical, ecological, and a gold mine of culinary possibilities. This chapter will help you make the best use of your machine and will answer the most frequently asked questions about grain cooking in a steamer.

Identifying Your Grain Steamer

Before you can understand how your grain steamer works, you must identify which type you own. As described in chapter 3, grain steamers come in two basic types: metal steamers and plastic steamers.

Metal steamers are easy to identify: they are round and the rice bowl is made of metal. Metal steamers have generally been used solely to steam rice. Until recently, they have been most commonly found in Asian restaurants or institutional settings. They are simple machines consisting of a heating element and a metal pot, a lid, and sometimes an on/off switch. Couldn't get much simpler.

Plastic steamers are equally easy to identify: they are round or oval with a rice bowl and housing made of plastic. Plastic steamers have a separate water reservoir that produces steam.

Troubleshooting

Know Your Machine

Q: What should I do if the timer goes off and my dish is not done cooking?

A: If you have a plastic machine, reset the timer for the amount of extra cooking time you think is needed. Usually it is best to add just 5–10 minutes at a time. See the chart in chapter 5.

If you have a metal machine, push the "warm" button back down to the "cook" position. You may need to add more water as well.

Q: Is it OK to take the lid off while the grain is cooking?

A: It is best to leave the lid on because each time you open it, steam escapes, thus extending the cooking time needed. Also you will risk burning yourself on the hot steam that will come pouring out from under the lid and from the machine.

Q: I bought a metal unit and it looks more like a Crock-Pot than a steamer. How does this steam foods?

A: Some machines come with a perforated insert which allows you to steam vegetables. Grains, on the other hand, do not require an insert. The grain is simply cooked by the hot steam which rises up, making small tunnels in the cooking grain for the steam to escape through. That is why it is best to avoid stirring the grain while it is cooking. Stirring destroys the tunnels, causing the grain to trap moisture and become sticky.

Q: What accessories can be purchased to be used in my metal steamer?

A: The collapsible stainless steel or plastic steamer baskets work well and come in many sizes. Plastic, rubber, or wooden spatulas make great serving utensils.

Cooking Tips

Q: How can I use my machine to reheat foods?

A: Both the metal and the plastic units can be used to heat up leftovers. The metal units may need a little water added to the bottom of the pan, or use the steamer insert and steam the food until warm. The plastic units will add plenty of moisture, so you may not need to add any liquid to the dish itself.

Q: What is the best way to prevent grains from sticking to the bottom of my steamer?

A: First, avoid using metal utensils in the machine. Either use the plastic spatula that came with the machine or buy a soft rubber spatula or plastic spoon. If you keep the plastic machines free of scratches, they virtually never have a sticking problem. If you already have done the damage and have a few scratches, liberally applying a nonstick oil spray may help reduce the problem. Also, if you let the water level get too low in the metal machine, you may get some sticking. So keep it moist; add water if you plan to keep a dish warm for a long period of time.

Machine Maintenance

Q: How should I clean my machine?

A: The metal steamers have an inner pot that slides out of its housing and can be cleaned with a scrub brush or sponge. The plastic units have plastic steamer bowls. These usually just need to be rinsed well; use a soft sponge so as not to scratch the plastic. You may need to use soap if there is an oil or fat residue.

Have you ever noticed how much easier the cleanup is after preparing a dish which has no fat? Just one more reason to reduce fat in our cooking.

Q: Can I use my dishwasher for my grain machine?

A: The plastic lid and bowls of most plastic machines can go on the top rack of the dishwasher, where they won't get so hot that they warp or melt. The metal units have a pan that slips out and can be washed in a machine.

Q: The plastic steamer bowls of my machine are becoming discolored. How can I clean them?

A: Many spices will discolor plastic because it is a porous material by nature. Turmeric and saffron colors plastic an attractive neon yellow, beets may dye your plastic pink, and berries also can tint plastic. You can use a dilute bleach solution to soak the plastic. Immerse the parts for an hour, then use soap to clean them and let them air dry overnight before cooking in them again.

Q: How can I properly dry my machine so that it isn't moist all the time and growing questionable little microbes?

A: After rinsing and while the unit may still be warm, keep the lid off and let it dry out in the air before putting it away in the cupboard.

Kitchen Science

Q: What can I do to make my grains come out softer and more tender?

A: First, if you are using salt in the recipe, add it at the end. Cooking grains with salt can make them tough. Next, use a little more cooking water and extend your cooking time by 5 minutes for every tablespoon of water.

Q: How can I get my rice to come out fluffy?

A: Rinsing the grain in cold water prior to cooking washes away some of the loose starch and results in fluffier rice.

Q: How can I get my rice to come out stickier for making rice balls?

A: Not rinsing the rice and adding slightly more water than normal will help the rice stick together. Short grain rice is naturally stickier than long grain.

Q: Why do the cooking time and water requirement vary even for rice?

A: Rice grains vary in size and water content. The older the grain, the dryer it is and the longer the cooking time and greater the cooking water requirement. Altitude affects boiling temperature and therefore also slightly affects cooking time.

Q: What is the ecological advantage to grain cookers?

A: These machines use very little energy compared to electric or gas ovens and stoves.

Q: Is there a nutritional advantage to using grain cookers?

A: Yes, steamers allow more control in using the minimal amount of steaming time, which saves nutrients such as water-soluble vitamins from being lost in overcooking. Also there is no frying involved, which causes denaturing of proteins and fats and has adverse health effects. With the plastic machines there is no charring, which is carcinogenic. Steaming foods helps them retain moisture, and moist foods are easier on the digestive system.

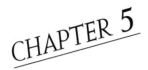

CHAPTER 5

In Search of the Perfect Grain

*H*alf the fun of owning a grain steamer is the joy of creating new recipes and discovering new flavors, aromas, and textures. Each set of recipes in the grain chapters begins with a basic grain recipe. Refer to those chapters for instructions on how to cook specific grains. The purpose of this chapter is to provide you with some basic buying and cooking skills and introduce some multigrain recipes, sauces, and accompaniments. If you run into trouble developing your own recipes or following ours, just turn to the Troubleshooting section in chapter 4.

Cooking Tips

These few tips will help to turn grain novices into grain gourmets.

- Rinse the raw grain in cold water if it looks dirty or you see foreign particles. If you have purchased your grain from a bin, it is a good idea to rinse your grains well.

- Add spices in whole form to the cooking water for flavored rice—for example, peppercorns, cinnamon sticks, cloves, and bay leaves for an Indian pilaf.
- Use vegetable broth instead of water when cooking grains. They will absorb the broth and be full of flavor. This is especially nice with rice, barley, and other plain grains. Wine can also be added to grains in place of some of the cooking liquid.

Shopping Tips

Here are a few things to remember when you go to the store to stock your grain pantry.

- Buy natural ingredients whenever possible. For example, some soy sauce products contain MSG (monosodium glutamate), which is allergenic for many people. They may also contain corn syrup, caramel coloring, sodium benzoate (which is frequently used as a preservative), and residues from chemical solvents. Fortunately, soy sauce can also be purchased in a natural form that has no artificial additives, and there are varieties now available in a low-sodium form.
- Buy organic whenever possible. Organic produce has not been treated or sprayed with any pesticides or fungicides. Our environment is contaminated enough already; give your body a break and buy pure foods. If your store does not carry organic foods, request them. Pester the management so that they understand there is a market for organic foods.
- Buy in bulk whenever possible. Bulk buying from a bin makes sense both economically and ecologically.
- Do not, however, buy from bulk bins if you have grain allergies or intolerances. The scoops in containers are easily cross-contaminated.
- Consider changing to soy milk. Soy milk is available in as wide a range of forms as cow's milk. There are lowfat and whole fat versions, malted, sweetened, flavored, or plain. Plain and vanilla are very nice on cereals. Soy milk contains

no lactose, cholesterol, or synthetic hormones, and when fortified is a vegetarian alternative to cow's milk. It is also loaded with beneficial phytochemicals.

Storage Tips

Whole grains have a higher oil content than refined grains because they contain the germ, so they must be protected against rancidity.

- Store grains in a cool, dry place, in a well-sealed container such as plastic or glass.
- Uncooked grains may be stored in the refrigerator or in the freezer, where they can last for years.
- Make sure that the storage container is tightly sealed. Bugs can find their way into grains even while left on the counter.
- Cooked grains can be stored in the refrigerator for almost a week.
- Freeze cooked grains for longer storage. Make sure to label the container with date and contents. Plastic freezer storage bags are what we use to store our own grains. We freeze them in meal-size batches so they are always on hand.

Presentation Tips

Grains are so versatile they can be presented in many different ways. You are limited only by your imagination. Here are some of our favorite presentations.

- Sticky grains such as cooked rice or cooked millet can be formed into balls and rolled in toasted sesame seeds.
- Whole cooked grains or grain dishes can be packed into a bread pan and sliced, then served with a drizzle of dressing or sauce.
- Medium- and short-grain rice and some of the smaller grains like quinoa and millet can be spooned into molds for a more

formal presentation. Use your small measuring cups as handy molds.

- Grains can be stuffed into vegetables such as peppers, tomatoes, eggplant, mushrooms, and apples.
- Sprinkle your favorite grains with fresh herbs. Fresh herbs can be purchased in the supermarket or grown at home.
- Use seasonings such as saffron and turmeric to color grains. These spices, when used in small amounts, will not change the flavor of a dish, but they will add an interesting color and important phytochemicals.

Organization Tips

Grain cooking is much easier with just a bit of preparation.

- Read the entire recipe before starting, to be sure you have the ingredients called for or appropriate substitutions.
- Do as much advance preparation as possible, such as cutting vegetables, chopping nuts, and roasting spices.
- Commonly used ingredients such as onions, garlic, and parsley can be chopped and stored in tightly covered plastic containers or bags.
- Put ingredients away after you have added what's needed to the recipe. This will free up counter space and remind you where you are within the recipe.
- Label all grains after cooking. It can be difficult to tell one berry from another.

Quick Grain Recipes

Here are some simple recipes that work well with most whole groats and berries. Use wheat, rye, triticale, spelt, Kamut berries, whole oat groats, or rice. Use cooked grains that have been stored in your refrigerator or freezer. With a plastic machine, add the minimum amount of water to the reservoir. For metal steamers, add an additional ½ cup of water to the rice bowl for each 1 cup of grain.

Raspberry Grain with Feta Cheese and Broccoli

1 cup chopped fresh broccoli or frozen broccoli
2 cups cooked grain
½ cup raspberry vinegar
¼ cup crumbled feta cheese

Add broccoli, brown rice, and vinegar to rice bowl. Steam for 15 minutes. Just before serving, sprinkle with feta cheese.

Serves 6

Carrot Rice with Peas and Peppers

2 cups cooked grain
½ cup pureed, steamed carrots
½ cup fresh or frozen peas
½ cup red pepper strips

Combine all ingredients in rice bowl and steam for 15 minutes.

Serves 6

Green, White, and Orange Grains

2 cups cooked grain
½ cup chopped kale
½ cup julienne carrots

Combine ingredients in rice bowl and steam for 15 minutes.

Serves 6

Milk Recipes

If you or your child suffers from a milk allergy, here are some alternatives to cows' milk that can be made at home. However, these are not nutritional substitutes for milk. Make sure you or your child has an adequate source of calcium and riboflavin in the diet.

Nut Milk

2 cups cold water
½ cup any type of nut (almonds and cashews work well)

Add ingredients to a blender and process until smooth. Strain off the nut sludge at the bottom (which incidentally is delicious on salads), and the milky fluid now left is wonderful on cereal. It can be used in place of dairy milk for any recipe, and is wheat-, lactose-, hormone-, and cholesterol-free. However, these milks are high in calories—heart-healthy calories, but calories all the same.

Makes 2½ cups

Oat Milk

1 cup whole oats
10 cups water
⅓ cup brown rice syrup or honey

Cook oats until mushy. Pour the mixture into a blender and purée. Strain the oat milk for a smoother-textured liquid and add sweetener. This grain milk is fairly low in fat, contains no cholesterol, and serves as a versatile dairy milk substitute.

Makes 10 to 11 cups

Grain Puddings

Who can resist the sweet, comforting taste of grain puddings? If you have eaten only rice puddings, your taste buds are in for a major treat.

1½ cups cooked grain
2 cups milk of your choice
¼ to ½ cup liquid sweetener

Options (singly or in combination):
½ teaspoon vanilla extract
½ teaspoon almond extract
½ cup chopped dried fruit such as cranberries, raisins, date pieces, prunes
Spices such as ½ teaspoon cinnamon, ½ teaspoon grated lemon or orange rind, ¼ teaspoon ground nutmeg or ginger
½ cup fresh fruit such as blueberries or strawberries
3 eggs, beaten, to give a more custard-like texture

Combine all ingredients in a 4-cup baking dish and stir to mix. Bake in a preheated 300° oven for 45 minutes or until set, stirring once after 15 minutes. Let sit for 10 minutes after baking, to set further. Serve hot or cold.

Makes 5½ cups

Multigrain Cereals

If you love variety in the morning, these multigrain mixes are for you. Just store them in sealed containers or bags until ready to cook.

Three Grain Cereal

½ cup rolled thick oats
½ cup rolled wheat or triticale
½ cup rolled rye
½ cup raisins
½ cup sunflower seeds
2 teaspoons apple pie spice
1 teaspoon salt (optional)

Combine ingredients and store in ¼-cup servings. See page 110 for cooking instructions.

Makes 10 ½-cup servings (cooked)

Four Grain Cereal

¾ cup rolled oats
¾ cup rolled rye
¾ cup rolled barley
¾ cup rolled wheat
¾ cup chopped dried apple
2 to 3 teaspoons cinnamon
½ teaspoon salt (optional)

Combine ingredients and store in ¼-cup servings. See page 110 for cooking instructions.

Makes 15 ½-cup servings (cooked)

Five Grain Cereal

½ cup steel-cut oats
½ cup cracked rye
½ cup brown rice farina
½ cup cracked wheat

¼ cup quinoa
¼ cup ground flaxseed
¼ cup slightly ground sunflower seeds
2 teaspoons pumpkin pie spice or cinnamon
1 teaspoon salt (optional)

Combine ingredients and store in ¼-cup servings. See page 159 for cooking instructions.

Makes 11 ½-cup servings (cooked)

Baby Cereals

For Babies Under Six Months

Brown rice makes the perfect first choice for a cereal because it is one of the least allergenic (allergy causing) grains. Ask your pediatrician when your infant should start solid foods.

¼ cup well-cooked brown rice
¼ cup breast milk or formula

Place ingredients in a blender or food processor and process until smooth. Refrigerate until needed.

Makes 2 ¼-cup servings

For Babies Six Months and Older

Avoid wheat grains during the first year. Barley, rice, and rye are good choices.

½ cup well-cooked grain
½ cup breast milk, formula, water, or juice

Place ingredients in a blender or food processor and process until smooth. Refrigerate until needed.

Makes 1 cup

For Babies over One Year

Any cereal you are making for the rest of the family can be given to older babies and toddlers. Avoid recipes that are very spicy or that contain small nuts that could get caught in the throat.

Alternate Cooking Instructions

Haven't bought a grain steamer yet? Just follow the instructions below.

1. Rinse grains under cold water to remove surface starch and debris.
2. Bring liquid to a boil in a heavy saucepan with a tight-fitting lid.
3. Add grains and heat to boiling again.
4. If you are cooking rice or millet, let grains cook for 15 minutes before adding any salt. (Salt increases the cooking time of these grains.)
5. Reduce heat and simmer for the recommended time, being careful not to remove the lid. For chewy grains, cook a few minutes less. For a softer grain, cook for a few minutes longer.
6. Add additional water if the grain is not cooked when all the liquid is absorbed.
7. To toast rice, bulgur, or buckwheat, put grains in a saucepan (ungreased), place over medium heat, and stir until grains deepen in color. Add liquid and cook as usual.
8. You may make enough grains to last the week and store them in the refrigerator.

Vitamin C–Containing Foods

Grains can be an excellent source of minerals, particularly iron. However, the phytic acid in the grains can prevent the absorption of some of these nutrients. When vitamin C is eaten at the same meal, it counteracts the phytic acid and increases the bioavailability of iron and other minerals from the grains. It's easy to add vitamin C to your meals. Here are some of our favorite ideas.

The first number listed is the milligrams of vitamin C per 100 grams of food (100 grams = 3½ ounces). This is followed by the food name and suggestions for incorporating it into your diet.

369 *Peppers, red chili*   Add small amounts to hot grain dishes.

190 *Peppers, red sweet*   Sweet and crunchy, these are great in salads and hot dishes. Roast them, peel off the skin, and purée into a *coulis* sauce to pour over grain and vegetable dishes or millet patties.

186 *Kale leaves*   Replace lettuce with kale for more fiber, minerals, and vitamin C.

172 *Parsley*   Fresh and finely chopped, this is a versatile herb especially important in pilafs and salads.

152 *Collard greens*   Great steamed alone with just a drizzle of lemon and butter or chopped fine in a pilaf recipe.

128 *Peppers, green sweet*   Cheap and available year round, these are a staple source of vitamin C for many households.

113 *Broccoli*   Slice the stalks for funky shapes kids love and serve steamed alone as a garnish. Also great with lemon.

102 *Brussels sprouts*   Steam them alone and toss into fluffy grain dishes for a fun presentation.

97 *Mustard greens*   Slice into long, thin strips, add a splash of vinegar, and use as a bed for grain dishes.

79 *Watercress*   Chopped fine, these little leaves can be slipped into any savory grain dish.

78 *Cauliflower*   Steam and blend with tomato sauce for an iron rich sauce.

66 *Persimmons*   Serve slices as a garnish for summer dishes.

61 *Red cabbage*   Slice whole rounds and steam, then layer a grain dish with several slices for a colorful presentation.

59 *Strawberries*   Add whole strawberries to breakfast cereal or purée to drizzle over rice farina.

56 *Papayas*   Slices with fresh lime juice are perfect as an accompaniment to breakfast cereals or as dessert to dinner dishes.

51 *Spinach*   Steamed or raw, chopped or sliced, use several leaves under a scoop of your favorite grain pilaf or salad.

50 *Oranges and their juice*   Have a piece of fruit or glass of juice with your breakfast cereal.

47 *Cabbage*   Chopped and mixed with lowfat yogurt, this is a cool side dish to serve with hot, spicy grain dishes.

46 *Lemon juice*   Drizzle on salads and steamed vegetables or mix with vinegar for a no-fat salad dressing to splash on cold grain dishes.

38 *Grapefruit and its juice*   Serve along with breakfast cereal.

36 *Turnips*   Slice thin and cook into hot grain dishes.

33 *Asparagus*   Steam it and served as a side dish to grain dishes.

33 *Cantaloupes*   Melon balls can be served on top of hot breakfast cereal or on the side.

32 *Swiss chard*   This can be steamed and served with lemon juice as a side dish.

28 *Lima beans, young*   Add a can of cooked beans to your favorite savory grain dish in the last 10 minutes of cooking time, to let them heat up. Also makes a complementary protein with grains.

29 *Black-eyed peas*   Traditionally served with collard greens in the south, they can be added to any savory grain dish.

29 *Soybeans*   Their creamy, rich texture adds a hearty element when puréed with sauces.

26 *Radishes*   Slice thinly and serve raw as a refreshing, crispy condiment.

25 *Raspberries*   Purée to serve as a spread or *coulis* over hot breakfast cereals.

25 *Chinese cabbage*   Also known as bok choy, is great raw or steamed. Chop 1 cup and toss with salads.

23   *Honeydew melon*   Can be made into melon balls or chopped and cooked into breakfast cereal as a sweetener.

23   *Tomatoes*   Whole stewed tomatoes, sauce, paste, cooked, or raw—there's an assortment of ways to add tomatoes to dishes. Chopping it fresh and adding it to pilafs and adding a few tablespoons of paste to grains dishes are our old standbys.

Guide to Water Amounts and Steaming Times for Plastic Machines

The cup amounts refer to the amount of water in the water reservoir. You can designate how long the machine steams by varying the amount of water. Water amounts and cooking times for the rice bowls differ, depending on the particular foods. See your manual for more information.

¼ cup	5–8 minutes	1½ cups	26–30 minutes
½ cup	9–11 minutes	1¾ cups	31–35 minutes
¾ cup	13–16 minutes	2 cups	36–41 minutes
1 cup	17–21 minutes	2½ cups	42–44 minutes
1¼ cups	22–25 minutes	3 cups	45–50 minutes

CHAPTER 6

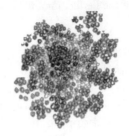

Amaranth (*Amaranthus cruentus*)

This tiny seed is creamy beige in color and has a woodsy flavor.

*F*irst cultivated by cave dwellers as early as 4000 B.C., amaranth had become as important a crop as corn and beans by the time of the Aztecs and Incas. It was a staple food of the Aztecs 500 years ago and was grown from what is now Arizona to Argentina. Amaranth was grown not only for its seeds but also for its delicious leaves. The Aztecs were producing an estimated fifteen to twenty thousand tons of amaranth leaves and seeds per year just prior to the Spanish conquest.

Amaranth was more than just a staple food to the Aztecs—it also played a symbolic role in Aztec religious ceremonies. Amaranth seeds were ground into a paste and then mixed with honey, out of which replicas of Aztec gods were fashioned. The edible figures were then fed to the worshippers. When Cortés invaded in 1519, he ordered the destruction of amaranth, because he considered the dough figures to be pagan shapes and suspected that human blood was mixed into the ceremonial dough. In order to discourage the Indians from growing amaranth, he threatened to cut off the hands of anyone who cultivated it.

As you might expect, amaranth production declined drastically, and wheat and corn replaced amaranth as staple grains. However, this self-seeding easy-to-grow plant managed to survive to modern times as a wild plant. In the last hundred years, amaranth grain has made steady gains, especially among Himalayan farmers. In India, where amaranth is known as *rajgira* (king seed) and *ramdana* (seed sent by god), the popped seeds are mixed with honey or syrup to make candy.

About 60 different species of amaranth are grown in Asia, Africa, and the Americas. Some are grown for food, some are grown as ornamentals, and others grow wild. The Rodale Research Center in Kutztown, Pennsylvania, is one of the leaders in the field of amaranth development.

What Is Amaranth?

Amaranth is not a true grain but the seed of a fast-growing, stress-resistant broadleaf plant. The amaranth is quite striking in appearance. It is tall, about the size of corn stalks, with brilliantly colored pinkish purple flower clusters that remain colored even when they are dried. The seeds are borne on spike-shaped heads that measure a foot or more in length and six inches across. There may be up to half a million seeds to a plant.

The amaranth seed is tiny, about the size of a grain of sand. The grain is covered with a tough seed coat; the uncooked seed is therefore not easily digested. Toasting or boiling the grain makes it chewable and digestible. The seeds have a mild, nutty flavor and can be used directly in breakfast cereals and granolas or ground into whole grain meal or flour for baking.

Nutrition and Amaranth

One cup of cooked amaranth supplies 276 mg of calcium, more than a quarter of the United States recommended daily allowance for that mineral. It also supplies over a third of the vitamin A and two-thirds of the vitamin E recommended each day. Nutritionally, it has over twice the amount of protein of corn and rice. What makes this grain so valuable, however, is its amino acid content. We mentioned that true cereal grains lack sufficient amounts of lysine but are good sources of leucine. Amaranth is a rich source of lysine and methionine but a poor source of leucine; therefore, amaranth makes a good protein complement to either grains or beans.

Amaranth is also a good source of dietary fiber, particularly insoluble fiber. Diets rich in insoluble fiber decrease the chances of developing constipation, diverticular disease, hemorrhoids, and varicose veins.

Health and Amaranth

Allergies

Amaranth is often called an ancient grain or a super grain. Because amaranth is not a true cereal grain and is not related to other grain families, it can often be tolerated by individuals with grain allergies.

Cancer

Amaranth is high in insoluble fiber, the kind of fiber that resists breakdown by both digestive enzymes and the bacterial enzymes of the colon. Diets rich in insoluble fiber are associated with lower risks of colon and rectal cancer.

Celiac Disease

Individuals who have celiac disease and are gluten intolerant should *not* eat amaranth. Amaranth is often portrayed as being essentially gluten free. This may be true, but until research proves that amaranth contains no amino acids that damage the intestinal linings of celiacs, it should be totally avoided by them.

High Cholesterol

Although it is low in soluble fiber, amaranth reduces high serum cholesterol levels just as pectin and oat bran do. This may be due to its high squalene content. Squalene is a lipid that is thought to reduce serum cholesterol by inhibiting HMG CoA reductase, the regulating enzyme for cholesterol synthesis.

Vegetarians

Amaranth complements the proteins found in other grains and legumes and increases the protein quality of the diet that does not contain animal protein. This makes it also valuable to individuals undergoing periods of growth, including young children, adolescents, and pregnant and lactating women.

How to Buy Amaranth

Amaranth grain can be purchased as a whole seed or as a flour. Look for seeds that are whole and do not smell of linseed. Such an odor means that the grain has become rancid. Amaranth can be purchased from specialty stores and health food stores. If you cannot locate amaranth in a store close to you, order it from one of the mail order companies listed in the back of the book.

How to Use Amaranth

Amaranth flour can be combined with high-gluten flours to make breads and other baked goods. Whole grain amaranth can be used as a porridge, combined with other grains in a pilaf, or added to baked grains. Amaranth has a long shelf life and is pest resistant.

Store the seeds in a sealed container and keep in a dry place.

Recipes

Basic Cooking Instructions

Rinse amaranth grains in water before cooking. Amaranth can be toasted for a nuttier taste. Just add the raw amaranth to a hot, unoiled skillet and stir until lightly browned. For breakfast grains, increase the amount of liquid in the rice bowl and substitute fruit juice for some or all of the cooking liquid. For dinner grains, substitute vegetable juice for some or all of the cooking liquid.

1 cup amaranth
1 cup water (juice or broth)
Salt to taste

Plastic Steamers

Fill water reservoir and turn on machine. Add ingredients to rice bowl and cover. Steam for 45 minutes.

Metal Steamers

Spray rice bowl with nonstick spray. Place ingredients in rice bowl and add an additional 1 cup of water (not juice or broth). Turn machine on. Remove grain from rice bowl before machine switches to warm, to prevent sticking. Set a timer for 45 minutes.

Serves 4

Breakfast Amaranth

A unique way to start the day. This recipe is sweet and warm: perfect for starting a winter day. This cereal is a rich source of calcium, iron, and protein.

1 cup water
¼ cup amaranth
½ cup pitted prunes, chopped
Lowfat milk or soy milk
Salt to taste

Plastic Steamers

Fill reservoir with water and turn on steamer. Add ingredients to rice bowl, cover, and steam for 45 minutes or until all liquid is absorbed. Add additional water to reservoir if necessary.

Metal Steamers

Coat rice bowl with nonstick spray and add ingredients. Add an additional 1 cup of water. Steam for 45 minutes or until liquid is almost absorbed. Add additional water to bowl if more cooking is necessary. Divide grain into 2 bowls and add milk. Serve warm.

Serves 2

Nutrition Facts

Serving Size 2.456 ounces (69.63g)
Servings Per Container 4

Amount Per Serving

Calories 59   Calories from Fat 2

	% Daily Value*
Total Fat 0g	0%
Saturated Fat 0g	0%
Cholesterol 0mg	0%
Sodium 11mg	0%
Total Carbohydrate 15g	5%
Dietary Fiber 6g	24%
Sugars 9g	
Protein 2g	

Vitamin A 17%	Vitamin C 35%
Calcium 11%	Iron 8%

*Percent Daily Values are based on a 2,000 calorie diet. Your daily values may be higher or lower depending on your calorie needs.

Hot Spicy Amaranth

A warm treat that is welcome any time of the day. However, we love it for breakfast.

2 cups water
1 cup amaranth seeds
¼ cup raisins
1 teaspoon cinnamon powder
⅛ teaspoon nutmeg powder
Shredded coconut for garnish

Plastic Steamers

Fill reservoir with water and turn on steamer. Add ingredients to rice bowl, cover, and steam for 45 minutes or until all liquid is absorbed. Add additional water to reservoir if necessary. Garnish with coconut if desired.

Metal Steamers

Coat rice bowl with nonstick spray and add ingredients. Add an additional 1 cup of water. Steam for 45 minutes or until liquid is almost absorbed. Add additional water to bowl if more cooking is necessary. Garnish with coconut if desired.

Serves 4

Nutrition Facts	
Serving Size 2.671 ounces (75.71g)	
Servings Per Container 4	
Amount Per Serving	
Calories 43 Calories from Fat 2	
	% *Daily Value**
Total Fat 0g	0%
Saturated Fat 0g	0%
Cholesterol 0mg	0%
Sodium 15mg	1%
Total Carbohydrate 10g	3%
Dietary Fiber 7g	28%
Sugars 6g	
Protein 2g	
Vitamin A 18%	Vitamin C 46%
Calcium 14%	Iron 10%

*Percent Daily Values are based on a 2,000 calorie diet. Your daily values may be higher or lower depending on your calorie needs.

Cold Amaranth Salad

Use this as a topping for a green salad. Try different vinegars—
our favorites are raspberry and balsamic.

⅛ cup cooked amaranth (use the basic amaranth recipe)
1 tablespoon red wine vinegar
2 teaspoons lemon juice
½ teaspoon light soy sauce

Mix ingredients together and serve as a salad topping, or multiply all the ingredients by 4 and you will have enough to
serve as a cold grain dish for two.

Serves 2

Nutrition Facts

Serving Size 2.825 ounces (80.08g)
Servings Per Container 2

Amount Per Serving

Calories 16   Calories from Fat 1

	% Daily Value*
Total Fat 0g	0%
Saturated Fat 0g	0%
Cholesterol 0mg	0%
Sodium 64mg	3%
Total Carbohydrate 4g	1%
Dietary Fiber 6g	24%
Sugars 0g	
Protein 1g	

Vitamin A 18%	Vitamin C 49%
Calcium 13%	Iron 8%

*Percent Daily Values are based on a
2,000 calorie diet. Your daily values
may be higher or lower depending on
your calorie needs.

Savory Amaranth

A fragrant, spicy accompaniment to chicken or fish.

1½ cups vegetable broth
1 cup amaranth seeds
2 teaspoons sesame oil
1 clove garlic, crushed
1 green onion, slivered
¼ cup diced red pepper
Soy sauce (optional)

Plastic Steamers
Fill reservoir with water and turn on steamer. Add ingredients to rice bowl, cover, and steam for 45 minutes or until all liquid is absorbed. Add additional water to reservoir if necessary. When amaranth is finished cooking, serve topped with a splash of soy sauce.

Metal Steamers
Coat rice bowl with nonstick spray and add ingredients. Add an additional 1 cup of water. Steam for 45 minutes or until liquid is almost absorbed. Add additional water to bowl if more cooking is necessary. When amaranth is finished cooking, serve topped with a splash of soy sauce.

Serves 4

Nutrition Facts	
Serving Size 6.320 ounces (179.2g)	
Servings Per Container 4	
Amount Per Serving	
Calories 51 Calories from Fat 20	
	% *Daily Value**
Total Fat 2g	3%
Saturated Fat 0g	0%
Cholesterol 3mg	1%
Sodium 168mg	6%
Total Carbohydrate 5g	2%
Dietary Fiber 7g	28%
Sugars 0g	
Protein 5g	
Vitamin A 19%	Vitamin C 54%
Calcium 14%	Iron 10%

*Percent Daily Values are based on a 2,000 calorie diet. Your daily values may be higher or lower depending on your calorie needs.

Spotted Rice

This side dish is good for introducing amaranth to the family. It is an excellent source of insoluble fiber and calcium. Vegetable juice or vegetable broth can be substituted for the chicken broth.

2 cups lowfat chicken broth
1½ cups long-grain brown rice
½ cup amaranth, toasted
¼ cup chopped fresh parsley
Salt and pepper

To toast amaranth: add raw grain to a hot, un-oiled skillet and heat until grain is a light golden brown. Be careful not to overcook.

Plastic Steamers
Fill reservoir with water and turn machine on. Add ingredients to rice bowl and cover. Steam for 45 minutes. Season and serve.

Metal Steamers
Coat rice bowl with nonstick cooking spray and add ingredients. Add an additional 1 cup of water to bowl. Cover and turn machine on. When machine turns off, let grain steam for an additional 10 minutes, then season and serve.

Serves 4

Nutrition Facts	
Serving Size 5.302 ounces (150.3g)	
Servings Per Container 4	
Amount Per Serving	
Calories 92 Calories from Fat 9	
	% *Daily Value**
Total Fat 1g	2%
Saturated Fat 0g	0%
Cholesterol 0mg	0%
Sodium 90mg	4%
Total Carbohydrate 18g	6%
Dietary Fiber 3g	12%
Sugars 0g	
Protein 3g	
Vitamin A 6%	Vitamin C 17%
Calcium 4%	Iron 6%

*Percent Daily Values are based on a 2,000 calorie diet. Your daily values may be higher or lower depending on your calorie needs.

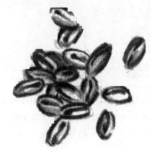

CHAPTER 7

Barley (Hordeum vulgare)

The whole barley grain has a sweet flavor and a resilient texture.

*B*arley is one of the oldest domesticated crops. It was an important food grain in prehistoric times, when it was probably used to make a porridge and as a base for fermented beverages. There was a type of barley used in settlements along the Nile as early as 18,300 years ago. The ancient Chinese viewed barley as a symbol of male potency because the heads of grain had heavy "beards" containing many seeds. In Greece, athletes ate a barley mush while in training because they believed it was easily digested. In Rome, barley was the special food of the gladiators, who were called *hordearii* or barley eaters. Barley was introduced by the Europeans to America, where it was first planted in 1602. It was probably grown for use in brewing.

Over the years, barley has been replaced by wheat and other grains; but today, it is still the fourth-ranking cereal food crop in the world. In America, barley is grown for human food, as fodder for animals, and as a source of enzymes and carbohydrate for brewing.

What Is Barley?

Barley is one of the cereal plants in the grass family. Its seeds grow in spikes or heads located at the tips of the stems. Like grains of oat and rye, the barley grain is a complete fruit that is covered by a tough, protective hull or husk. Like the wheat grain, the barley grain has an outer seed coat that covers the bran layer, a large starchy endosperm, and an oil-containing germ. The hull and bran are removed by a process called pearling.

Nutrition and Barley

Barley is an excellent source of polysaccharides. Besides being an excellent source of starch, barley contains beta-glucans and pentosans—often referred to as the "gum" component—and cellulose, the insoluble fiber component. It is the gum component of barley that is chiefly believed to reduce high serum cholesterol levels. Barley is also a source of potassium, magnesium, and niacin.

Health and Barley

High Cholesterol

Barley has been shown to lower cholesterol in individuals with high serum cholesterol levels. It contains three compounds which may be responsible.

- Barley is a rich source of beta-glucans which are associated with decreased cholesterol levels. Beta-glucans may achieve this by increasing thickness (viscosity) of intestinal contents.
- The bran found in hulled or hull-less unpearled barley contains tocotrienol, a form a vitamin E which may be able to prevent the liver from producing too much cholesterol.
- Barley is also rich in insoluble fiber, which may bind the cholesterol in the intestine and prevents its reabsorption.

Diabetes and Hypoglycemia

Barley has traditionally been used in the management of diabetes in Iraq. It has led to better control of diabetes with fewer complications. Researchers believe that the mineral chromium present in the barley is responsible. Chromium is a part of glucose tolerance factor, which helps the body to utilize glucose.

Immune Functioning

Barley appears to have some antiviral activity. The exact phytochemical responsible has not yet been identified; but if you are prone to colds in the winter, some barley added to hot soup may be in order.

How to Buy Barley

Barley comes in a variety of forms. It can be purchased in packages or from bulk bins. If you cannot purchase the type of barley you need at the supermarket or health food store, try the mail order companies in the back of this book.

Pearl Barley

Pearl barley is pearled, or milled, to remove the hull and the bran layers. This results in small round grains containing endosperm and little of the bran. Much of barley's protein, fiber, vitamins, and minerals are lost in the pearling process. Pearl barley is the equivalent of white rice, and we recommend that you purchase only hulled or hull-less barley.

Hulled Barley

Hulled barley, sometimes called pot barley, is barley that has been pearled only enough to remove the inedible hull. Most of the bran and germ layers are left intact.

Hull-less Barley

Hull-less barley is a new strain of barley with an easy-to-remove hull. This results in a groat that contains more of the bran layers than pearl barley.

Scotch Barley

Scotch barley is coarsely ground hulled barley. It can be added to soups or stews as a thickener or served hot as a porridge.

Rolled Barley

Rolled barley is pearl barley that is cut into slices, steamed, and then rolled into thin flakes. Rolled barley can be substituted for other rolled cereals.

How to Use Barley

Cook a week's worth of barley in your steamer and add it to bread recipes, soups, stews, stuffings, and pilafs. Cooked whole, it makes hearty cold salads. Blend cooked barley into a purée and add to soups to give a creamy, nonfat texture.

Store barley in a tightly closed container. It can be frozen for longer storage.

Recipes

Basic Cooking Instructions

Rinse barley grains in water before cooking. For breakfast grains, increase the amount of liquid in the rice bowl and substitute fruit juice for some or all of the cooking liquid. For dinner grains, substitute vegetable juice or broth for some or all of the cooking liquid. To decrease cooking time, soak grains overnight.

1 cup barley (presoaked)
1 cup water (juice or broth)
Salt to taste

Plastic Steamers
Fill water reservoir to the maximum and turn on machine. Add
ingredients to rice bowl and cover. Steam for 1 hour.

Metal Steamers
Spray rice bowl with nonstick spray. Place ingredients in rice
bowl and add an additional 1 cup of water (not juice or
broth). Turn machine on. Steam for 1 hour. Let grain steam on
warm for 10 minutes before serving.

Serves 4

Nutrition Facts

Serving Size 1.764 ounces (50.00g)
Servings Per Container 4

Amount Per Serving

Calories 174   Calories from Fat 5

	% Daily Value*
Total Fat 1g	2%
Saturated Fat 0g	0%
Cholesterol 0mg	0%
Sodium 0mg	0%
Total Carbohydrate 38g	13%
Dietary Fiber 0g	0%
Sugars 0g	
Protein 5g	

Vitamin A -%	Vitamin C -%
Calcium 1%	Iron 7%

*Percent Daily Values are based on a
2,000 calorie diet. Your daily values
may be higher or lower depending on
your calorie needs.

Breakfast Barley

A hearty breakfast cereal that is a perfect choice for individuals who have to watch their insulin levels. Barley and apples are good sources of the mineral chromium, which is a part of glucose tolerance factor. The cinnamon also increases glucose tolerance.

1 cup water
1 cup barley flakes
¼ cup chopped dried apple
2 tablespoons honey
1 teaspoon pumpkin pie spice
Salt to taste

Plastic Steamers
Fill reservoir with water and turn on steamer. Add ingredients to rice bowl and steam for 20 minutes or until done.

Metal Steamers
Coat rice bowl with nonstick spray and add ingredients, laying apple slices on top of cereal. Add an additional ¼ cup of water. Steam for 20 minutes or until machine turns off. Remove from pot immediately to prevent sticking.

Serves 4

Nutrition Facts	
Serving Size 1.457 ounces (41.30g)	
Servings Per Container 4	
Amount Per Serving	
Calories 134	Calories from Fat 3
	% *Daily Value**
Total Fat 0g	0%
Saturated Fat 0g	0%
Cholesterol 0mg	0%
Sodium 5mg	0%
Total Carbohydrate 32g	11%
Dietary Fiber 1g	4%
Sugars 9g	
Protein 2g	
Vitamin A 0%	Vitamin C 0%
Calcium 1%	Iron 4%

*Percent Daily Values are based on a 2,000 calorie diet. Your daily values may be higher or lower depending on your calorie needs.

Quick Barley Pilaf

Keep the ingredients on hand and this dish can be quickly prepared in a pinch. The perfect potluck or lunch box pleaser.

1 cup water
½ cup hulled or hull-less barley
½ cup medium brown rice
1 cup lowfat chicken broth
1 tablespoon dried onion
1 tablespoon dried parsley
½ teaspoon pepper

Plastic Steamers
In the morning, add water and
grains to rice bowl and let
grains soak until evening. Drain
barley and add to rice bowl. Fill
reservoir with water. Add remaining ingredients to rice
bowl and steam for 50 to 60
minutes.

Metal Steamers
In the morning, coat rice bowl
with nonstick spray, add water
and grains to rice bowl, and let
grains soak until evening. When
ready to cook, add remaining
ingredients without draining
grains. Turn on machine and
steam until steamer switches to
warm. Let pilaf steam on warm
setting for 10 minutes.

Serves 4

Nutrition Facts	
Serving Size 3.987 ounces (113.0g)	
Servings Per Container 4	
Amount Per Serving	
Calories 205 Calories from Fat 12	
	% *Daily Value**
Total Fat 1g	2%
Saturated Fat 0g	0%
Cholesterol 0mg	0%
Sodium 98mg	15%
Total Carbohydrate 44g	15%
Dietary Fiber 1g	4%
Sugars 0g	
Protein 6g	
Vitamin A 0%	Vitamin C 6%
Calcium 3%	Iron 10%

*Percent Daily Values are based on a
2,000 calorie diet. Your daily values
may be higher or lower depending on
your calorie needs.

Barley Raisin Salad

The barley can be made beforehand and stored, covered, in the refrigerator. This recipe also works well with brown rice, wheat berries, spelt, Kamut, or wild rice.

3 cups cooked barley (1 cup uncooked)
¼ cup raisins
¼ cup almonds, chopped
¼ cup celery, finely chopped
¼ cup carrot, grated
¼ cup onion, finely chopped

Dressing

2 ounces lemon juice
2 ounces olive oil
1 tablespoon tamari

Cook barley according to Basic Cooking Instructions. Let cool. Place in bowl and stir to fluff. Add remaining ingredients, dressing, and toss.

Serves 6

Nutrition Facts

Serving Size 3.101 ounces (87.92g)
Servings Per Container 6

Amount Per Serving

Calories 258 Calories from Fat 110

	% Daily Value*
Total Fat 12g	18%
Saturated Fat 2g	10%
Cholesterol 0mg	0%
Sodium 180mg	11%
Total Carbohydrate 35g	12%
Dietary Fiber 1g	4%
Sugars 1g	
Protein 5g	

Vitamin A 13%	Vitamin C 10%
Calcium 3%	Iron 8%

*Percent Daily Values are based on a 2,000 calorie diet. Your daily values may be higher or lower depending on your calorie needs.

Japanese Barley Rice

This simple recipe has a hearty bite and mild flavor. Miso paste comes in a plastic tub that keeps for several months in the refrigerator. Keep some on hand and this dish may become an old standby at your house.

1½ cups water
2 tablespoons miso paste
1 cup presoaked barley
½ cup short-grain brown rice
3 or 4 slices pickles (optional)
Fresh sliced ginger for garnish (optional)

Plastic Steamers
Fill reservoir with water and turn on steamer. Mix miso paste with a little water to dissolve it. Add ingredients to rice bowl and steam for 60 minutes or until done.

Metal Steamers
Coat rice bowl with nonstick spray. Add all ingredients to rice bowl with an additional 1 cup of water and cook for 60 minutes.

Serves 4

Nutrition Facts	
Serving Size 1.586 ounces (44.97g)	
Servings Per Container 4	
Amount Per Serving	
Calories 153 Calories from Fat 9	
	% *Daily Value**
Total Fat 1g	2%
Saturated Fat 0g	0%
Cholesterol 0mg	0%
Sodium 157mg	7%
Total Carbohydrate 32g	11%
Dietary Fiber 0g	0%
Sugars 0g	
Protein 4g	
Vitamin A 0%	Vitamin C 0%
Calcium 1%	Iron 5%

*Percent Daily Values are based on a 2,000 calorie diet. Your daily values may be higher or lower depending on your calorie needs.

Indian Spice Barley

This traditional Indian dish has incredible depth of flavor. The fragrance will fill the house with subtle scents of the East.

2½ cups water
1 cup hull-less barley
1 teaspoon ground cumin
½ teaspoon cardamom powder
2 bay leaves
½ teaspoon cinnamon powder
⅛ teaspoon clove powder
Salt to taste
2 tablespoons fresh chopped parsley

Plastic Steamers

In the morning, add water and barley to rice bowl and let grains soak until evening. Strain barley and add all ingredients except parsley. Fill reservoir with water. Steam for 60 minutes. When barley is tender, add parsley and serve.

Metal Steamers

In the morning, coat rice bowl with nonstick spray, add water and grains to rice bowl, and let grains soak until evening. Add all ingredients, except parsley. Turn on machine, add 1 extra cup of water, and steam until steamer switches to warm. Let dish steam on warm setting for 10 minutes. Add parsley and serve.

Serves 4

Nutrition Facts	
Serving Size 1.880 ounces (53.29g)	
Servings Per Container 4	
Amount Per Serving	
Calories 179 Calories from Fat 7	
	% *Daily Value**
Total Fat 1g	2%
Saturated Fat 0g	0%
Cholesterol 0mg	0%
Sodium 2mg	0%
Total Carbohydrate 39g	13%
Dietary Fiber 0g	0%
Sugars 0g	
Protein 5g	
Vitamin A 1%	Vitamin C 3%
Calcium 2%	Iron 11%

*Percent Daily Values are based on a 2,000 calorie diet. Your daily values may be higher or lower depending on your calorie needs.

Barley and Mushrooms

This recipe is also a modification of a traditional East Indian or Ayurvedic recipe. The ingredients are a thoughtful combination of herbs and spices for health and pleasure.

1 cup water
1 cup presoaked barley
½ cup mushrooms (shitake are very nice)
1 tablespoon butter or ghee (optional)
3 tablespoons fresh parsley, chopped fine
1 tablespoon sesame seeds
1 teaspoon mustard seeds
¼ teaspoon fresh ground black pepper
⅛ teaspoon clove powder
Salt to taste

Optional: Heat butter or ghee in pan and cook mustard seeds until they pop, then add to other ingredients in steamer bowl.

Plastic Steamers
Fill reservoir with water and turn on steamer. Add ingredients and steam for 60 minutes. Season and serve.

Metal Steamers
Coat rice bowl with nonstick spray, add ingredients and an additional cup of water. Cook until machine turns off and steam on warm for 10 minutes. Season and serve.

Serves 4

Nutrition Facts	
Serving Size 0.537 ounces (15.22g)	
Servings Per Container 4	

Amount Per Serving	
Calories 21 Calories from Fat 13	

	% *Daily Value**
Total Fat 1g	2%
Saturated Fat 0g	0%
Cholesterol 0mg	0%
Sodium 3mg	0%
Total Carbohydrate 2g	1%
Dietary Fiber 1g	4%
Sugars 0g	
Protein 1g	

Vitamin A 1%	Vitamin C 5%
Calcium 3%	Iron 4%

*Percent Daily Values are based on a 2,000 calorie diet. Your daily values may be higher or lower depending on your calorie needs.

Barley and Broccoli

A combination of two great chromium sources. A dish that all individuals who have diabetes or hypoglycemia should eat regularly.

1 cup hull-less barley, soaked
½ cup water
6 ounces chicken or vegetable broth
1 cup frozen or fresh chopped broccoli
¼ cup chopped cilantro
Salt to taste

Plastic Steamers

Fill reservoir with water and turn on steamer. Add barley, water, and broth to rice bowl. Steam for 50 minutes, add broccoli, and steam until broccoli is tender. Add cilantro, season, and serve.

Metal Steamers

Coat rice bowl with nonstick spray and add barley, water, broth, and an additional 1 cup of water. Steam until machine turns off, add broccoli, and steam on warm until broccoli is tender. Add cilantro, season, and serve.

Serves 4

Nutrition Facts	
Serving Size 4.772 ounces (135.3g)	
Servings Per Container 4	

Amount Per Serving	
Calories 191 Calories from Fat 8	

	% *Daily Value**
Total Fat 1g	2%
Saturated Fat 0g	0%
Cholesterol 0mg	0%
Sodium 75mg	3%
Total Carbohydrate 41g	14%
Dietary Fiber 1g	4%
Sugars 1g	
Protein 7g	

Vitamin A 7%	Vitamin C 54%
Calcium 4%	Iron 11%

*Percent Daily Values are based on a 2,000 calorie diet. Your daily values may be higher or lower depending on your calorie needs.

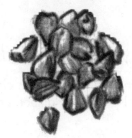

CHAPTER 8

Buckwheat (*Fagopyrum esculentum*)

Hulled, toasted buckwheat, or kasha, is reddish brown in color and has a robust, earthy flavor.

*B*uckwheat is a native of central Asia and was brought to Europe by the end of the Middle Ages, perhaps by the crusaders. It was sometimes called Saracen corn or wheat. Common buckwheat was cultivated widely in China as early as A.D. 900. Today, Russians eat buckwheat as a kind of boiled mush or porridge called kasha.

What Is Buckwheat?

Buckwheat is not a form of wheat, or even a relative of wheat. It is technically not even a grain but is instead an annual that is related to dock and rhubarb. The buckwheat plant is a small bushlike herb with smooth succulent leaves. It produces a pale three-cornered seed that is covered by a tough protective hull. It thrives on poor soil and an inhospitable climate.

Unlike other grains which are brown after hulling, buckwheat is cream colored. Brown buckwheat or kasha gets its color from roasting.

Hulled buckwheat has a bland flavor. It easily assimilates the flavors with which it is cooked. When roasted, the kernels take on a distinctive earthy taste.

Nutrition and Buckwheat

Buckwheat is higher in protein than most other grains. The protein is also higher in lysine, the amino acid in limited supply in true cereal grains. One cup of buckwheat supplies approximately a quarter of the day's magnesium and manganese and is also a good source of copper and niacin.

Even though buckwheat is not a true cereal grain, it does contains a small amount of gluten. This makes it unsuitable for individuals who are celiacs or gluten sensitive.

Health and Buckwheat

Cancer

Buckwheat is an excellent source of rutin, a flavonoid. Flavonoids are phytochemicals that act as antioxidants and protect the body's tissues from free-radical damage. Free-radical damage has been linked to cancer and heart disease. While there has been no research done on buckwheat and cancer, it seems prudent to include this nutritious grain as part of a healthful diet.

Vegetarians

Buckwheat contains more of the amino acid lysine than the true cereal grains. For individuals who eat little or no animal products, buckwheat can increase the quality of protein in the diet.

Wheat Allergy

Because buckwheat is *not* a relative of wheat, it is a good choice for people who suffer from wheat allergies. Buckwheat makes an excellent breakfast cereal and dinner pilaf.

How to Buy Buckwheat

Buckwheat is available in health food stores and by mail order. An increasing number of supermarkets also stock this grain. Buckwheat is available in packages and in bulk. There are two basic types.

White Buckwheat

White buckwheat is hulled buckwheat. The grain is passed between two millstones and the hull is cracked without grinding the seed. It is bland in flavor and easily takes on the flavors of foods and seasonings it is prepared with. If you have tasted buckwheat and have not liked the flavor, chances are you have tasted *kasha* which is toasted buckwheat. Give this nutritious grain another chance and try white buckwheat. It can replace rice in almost any recipe. White whole buckwheat is sold as whole groats or as stone-ground grits. Fine grind buckwheat makes an excellent breakfast porridge. White buckwheat can be pan roasted to make kasha.

Kasha

Kasha is buckwheat groats that have been hulled, crushed, and then toasted until they develop a deep brown color and a distinctive earthy flavor. Kasha is available in several grind sizes. Whole buckwheat or coarse grinds are good for pilafs and dinner grains.

How to Use Buckwheat

Buckwheat can be used in pilafs, as dinner grains, and as a breakfast porridge. Kasha makes a different and tasty addition to soups. Because of its hearty taste, kasha is a great choice for a dinner entrée. Buckwheat is one of the quickest cooking of all the grains. When made in the steamer, buckwheat cooks up light and fluffy with no mushiness.

Like all whole grains, buckwheat should be stored in a tightly closed container and in a cool, dark place.

Recipes

Basic Cooking Instructions

Buckwheat is a very quick cooking grain, so keep a close watch the first few times you prepare it. Wash buckwheat quickly and carefully. It is very porous and will absorb water readily. Buckwheat prepared in the steamer cooks up fluffy and separate. If the groats are too mushy, reduce cooking time or the amount of water in the rice bowl.

Kasha is traditionally cooked by first sealing the groat with egg: 1 to 2 cups of buckwheat are stirred with a beaten egg. The egg-coated groats are then roasted in a shallow pan until the kernels are dry, about 3 minutes. Steam as usual.

Nutrition Facts	
Serving Size 1.446 ounces (41.00g)	
Servings Per Container 4	
Amount Per Serving	
Calories 142 Calories from Fat 10	
	% *Daily Value**
Total Fat 1g	2%
Saturated Fat 0g	0%
Cholesterol 0mg	0%
Sodium 4mg	0%
Total Carbohydrate 31g	10%
Dietary Fiber 3g	12%
Sugars 0g	
Protein 5g	
Vitamin A 0%	Vitamin C 0%
Calcium 0%	Iron 5%

*Percent Daily Values are based on a 2,000 calorie diet. Your daily values may be higher or lower depending on your calorie needs.

1 cup white or roasted buckwheat
1 cup water, broth, or juice
Salt to taste

Plastic Steamers
Fill water reservoir and turn on machine. Add ingredients to
rice bowl and cover. Steam for a scant 5 minutes.

Metal Steamers
Spray rice bowl with nonstick spray. Place ingredients in rice
bowl and steam on warm, not on, for 6 minutes.

Serves 4

Breakfast Buckwheat

A very quick cooking breakfast with an unusual texture.

⅔ cup soy milk or cow's milk
½ cup white buckwheat
1 tablespoon molasses
⅛ teaspoon salt

Plastic Steamers
Add minimum amount of water
to reservoir and turn on machine. Add all ingredients to
rice bowl and steam for 5
minutes.

Metal Steamers
Coat rice bowl with nonstick
spray. Add ingredients to rice
bowl and steam on warm, not
on, for 6 to 7 minutes.

Serves 4

Nutrition Facts	
Serving Size 3.100 ounces (87.89g)	
Servings Per Container 4	
Amount Per Serving	
Calories 181 Calories from Fat 20	
	% *Daily Value**
Total Fat 2g	3%
Saturated Fat 0g	0%
Cholesterol 0mg	0%
Sodium 25mg	1%
Total Carbohydrate 37g	12%
Dietary Fiber 5g	20%
Sugars 0g	
Protein 7g	
Vitamin A 8%	Vitamin C 0%
Calcium 9%	Iron 11%

*Percent Daily Values are based on a 2,000 calorie diet. Your daily values may be higher or lower depending on your calorie needs.

Buckwheat Pilaf

A great change of pace from rice or potatoes. This is a quick cooking choice for those days when dinner must be made in a hurry.

1 cup white buckwheat
1 cup lowfat chicken broth
⅔ cup chopped green onions
2 tablespoons cider vinegar
⅛ teaspoon pepper

Plastic Steamers
Fill water reservoir with minimum quantity of water and turn machine on. Add ingredients to rice bowl and steam for 5 minutes.

Metal Steamers
Coat rice bowl with nonstick spray and add ingredients to rice bowl. Cook on warm, not on, for 6 minutes.

Serves 4

Nutrition Facts	
Serving Size 3.833 ounces (108.7g)	
Servings Per Container 4	
Amount Per Serving	
Calories 152 Calories from Fat 16	
	% *Daily Value**
Total Fat 2g	3%
Saturated Fat 0g	0%
Cholesterol 0mg	0%
Sodium 84mg	4%
Total Carbohydrate 31g	10%
Dietary Fiber 5g	20%
Sugars 0g	
Protein 7g	
Vitamin A 0%	Vitamin C 1%
Calcium 0%	Iron 6%

*Percent Daily Values are based on a 2,000 calorie diet. Your daily values may be higher or lower depending on your calorie needs.

Kasha

This is a variation of a traditional savory kasha recipe. It's very unusual to our Western palates—and who knows, you just might love it.

Egg wash:

1 raw egg white
½ cup water

Kasha:

1 cup kasha
2 cups chopped onion, sautéed
½ cup white wine
1 teaspoon dried thyme
1 teaspoon celery seeds
¼ teaspoon ground cinnamon

Plastic Steamers
Fill reservoir with minimum amount of water and turn on. Mix egg with water by whipping well, then coat kasha with this mixture. Pour into steamer bowl along with rest of ingredients and stir. Steam for 5 to 17 minutes and serve.

Nutrition Facts	
Serving Size 5.638 ounces (159.8g)	
Servings Per Container 4	
Amount Per Serving	
Calories 200 Calories from Fat 13	
	% *Daily Value**
Total Fat 1g	2%
Saturated Fat 0g	0%
Cholesterol 0mg	0%
Sodium 23mg	1%
Total Carbohydrate 39g	13%
Dietary Fiber 4g	16%
Sugars 2g	
Protein 7g	
Vitamin A 0%	Vitamin C 8%
Calcium 4%	Iron 11%

*Percent Daily Values are based on a 2,000 calorie diet. Your daily values may be higher or lower depending on your calorie needs.

Metal Steamers
Coat rice bowl with nonstick spray. Mix egg with water by whipping well, then coat kasha with this mixture. Pour into steamer bowl along with rest of ingredients and stir. Steam for 10 minutes and serve.

Serves 4

Kasha Southwest Salad

Here's a new twist to an old recipe. Enjoy this spicy combination with cornbread for a hearty winter meal.

1 tablespoon olive oil
¾ cup minced yellow onion
¼ cup diced celery
½ cup diced carrot
2 cloves garlic, minced
1 tablespoon diced jalapeno (discard seeds)
2½ cups cooked kasha
1½ teaspoons ground cumin
1½ teaspoons ground coriander
1 teaspoon chili powder
1 cup cooked or canned kidney beans, drained
¾ cup coarsely chopped tomato
¼ cup cooked corn kernels
1 cup spicy salsa
2 tablespoons chopped parsley
2 tablespoons chopped cilantro

Plastic Steamers

Add minimum amount of water
to reservoir and turn machine
on. Heat oil in sauce pan and
add onion, celery, carrot, garlic,
and jalapeno peppers. Sauté for
5 minutes. Add this mixture to
steamer, along with cumin, coriander, and chili powder. Steam
for 10 to 15 minutes. When
vegetables are cooked, add
kasha, beans, tomato, corn,
salsa, parsley, and cilantro. Mix
and serve.

Nutrition Facts	
Serving Size 8.576 ounces (243.1g)	
Servings Per Container 6	
Amount Per Serving	
Calories 175 Calories from Fat 31	
	% *Daily Value**
Total Fat 3g	5%
Saturated Fat 1g	5%
Cholesterol 1mg	0%
Sodium 369mg	23%
Total Carbohydrate 32g	11%
Dietary Fiber 5g	20%
Sugars 1g	
Protein 7g	
Vitamin A 59%	Vitamin C 43%
Calcium 4%	Iron 15%

*Percent Daily Values are based on a
2,000 calorie diet. Your daily values
may be higher or lower depending on
your calorie needs.

Metal Steamers

Coat rice bowl with nonstick spray and add 1 cup of additional water. Heat oil in sauce pan and add onion, celery, carrot, garlic, and jalapeno peppers. Sauté for 5 minutes. Add cumin, coriander, and chili powder. Add this mixture to kasha and cook in rice steamer for 10 to 15 minutes. When vegetables are cooked, add beans, tomato, corn, parsley, salsa, and cilantro. Mix and serve.

Serves 6

Tomato Buckwheat Sauce

This sauce makes reheated brown rice or noodles a nutritious meatless entrée.

1 cup white buckwheat
1 15-ounce can stewed tomatoes, Italian style
1 medium onion, cut into
    thin rings
2 cloves garlic, chopped

Plastic Steamers

Fill water reservoir to minimum level and turn on machine. Add ingredients and steam for 5 minutes. Sautéing onions and garlic first will increase flavor.

Metal Steamers

Coat rice bowl with nonstick spray and add ingredients. Cook on warm, not on, for 6 minutes. Sautéing onions and garlic first will increase flavor.

Serves 4

Nutrition Facts	
Serving Size 6.755 ounces (191.5g)	
Servings Per Container 4	

Amount Per Serving	
Calories 189 Calories from Fat 15	
	% Daily Value*
Total Fat 2g	3%
Saturated Fat 0g	0%
Cholesterol 0mg	0%
Sodium 325mg	14%
Total Carbohydrate 41g	14%
Dietary Fiber 6g	24%
Sugars 1g	
Protein 7g	

Vitamin A 7%	Vitamin C 31%
Calcium 5%	Iron 10%

*Percent Daily Values are based on a 2,000 calorie diet. Your daily values may be higher or lower depending on your calorie needs.

Buckwheat Salad

A filling, lowfat lunch time alternative.

3 cups buckwheat, cooked, chilled
1 cup lowfat cottage cheese
¼ cup barbecue sauce
3 cups chopped romaine lettuce

Prepare buckwheat according to Basic Cooking Instructions.
Toss with cottage cheese and sauce. Chill. Serve over bed of
romaine lettuce.

Serves 3

Nutrition Facts

Serving Size 9.264 ounces (262.6g)
Servings Per Container 4

Amount Per Serving

Calories 206   Calories from Fat 21

	% Daily Value*
Total Fat 2g	3%
Saturated Fat 1g	5%
Cholesterol 5mg	2%
Sodium 366mg	15%
Total Carbohydrate 35g	12%
Dietary Fiber 4g	16%
Sugars 5g	
Protein 14g	

Vitamin A 13%	Vitamin C 18%
Calcium 6%	Iron 10%

*Percent Daily Values are based on a
2,000 calorie diet. Your daily values
may be higher or lower depending on
your calorie needs.

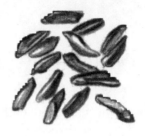

CHAPTER 9

Kamut (*Triticum polonicum*)

Whole kernels resemble large, golden grains of rice with a distinguishing hump. They have a rich, buttery flavor and chewy texture.

Kamut may date back as far as six thousand years. In Portugal in 1949, a U.S. airman from Montana was given thirty-six kernels of grain which were said to have come from an ancient tomb in the Nile valley near Dahshur in Egypt. The airman sent the kernels to his parents in Montana. Thirty-two of the kernels germinated, and within six years about fifteen hundred bushels were accumulated, drawing some attention as "King Tut's wheat." As the novelty diminished, the grain was forgotten.

In 1978 one jar of grains was rediscovered by Mack and Bob Quinn, who named the grain Kamut, the supposed ancient Egyptian word for wheat. In 1989 they released a premium organic Kamut to manufacturers and distributors in the natural foods industry. The Kamut seeds originally sent to Montana were not from an ancient Egyptian tomb—there are no reports of any viable wheat kernels surviving in ancient tombs—but it is undoubtedly an ancient wheat that originated in the Mediterranean area.

What Is Kamut?

Kamut (pronounced *Ka-moot*) is a nonhybrid cereal grain. A distant cousin to durum wheat, it is also related to spelt and common wheat. All three belong to the *Triticum* genus of cereal grasses.

Kamut looks like a giant soft, pale wheat grain with a humpback. It is easier to chew than wheat berries and has a soft, buttery flavor.

Nutrition and Kamut

Kamut is higher in protein, magnesium, and potassium than regular wheat and is a good source of the B vitamins folacin, thiamin, and niacin. Because the grain is so large, there is a greater percentage of endosperm relative to bran coating, which makes the whole grain more acceptable to people who are used to refined grains.

Health and Kamut

Allergies

Because it is an ancient strain of wheat that is not hybridized, Kamut may be tolerated by some people with wheat allergies. There is very little medical evidence to prove that Kamut is nonallegenic, but a great deal of anecdotal information. If you suffer from severe allergies, introduce Kamut into your diet only under a physician's supervision.

Celiac Disease

Kamut, like wheat, contains gluten. It must be totally avoided by those with gluten sensitivities such as celiac disease.

How to Buy Kamut

Kamut is not yet widely available. It can be found in some health food stores. It may be easier and faster to order through the mail from the companies listed in the back of the book. Kamut is also available in a very limited variety of forms. If you would like to try grinding your own Kamut into smaller grinds, purchase a grain mill at your local health food store.

Kamut Flour

Kamut flour can be used in all recipes as a replacement for wheat flour. It can be substituted for wheat flour in steamed pudding recipes.

Kamut Groats

Kamut is usually available as whole grain groats. These groats are all organically grown and contain all of the bran.

How to Use Kamut

Kamut can be substituted for wheat in any recipe. Use whole Kamut groats in pilafs, stuffings, soups, and stews. It can be served cold in salads. Kamut should be stored in a cool, dry place in a tightly sealed container.

Recipes

Basic Cooking Instructions

Like wheat and spelt, Kamut groats are very hard. They will cook faster if presoaked.

1 cup Kamut groats
1 cup water, juice, or broth
Salt to taste

Plastic Steamers

Add 1 cup of water to rice bowl along with grain. Let soak overnight or during the day. When ready to cook, fill water reservoir to the maximum, drain Kamut, and add back 1 cup of water or other cooking liquid. Steam until groats are soft and chewy, 50 to 60 minutes. If you have not soaked the grain, your cooking time will be closer to 90 minutes.

Metal Steamers

Coat rice bowl with nonstick spray. Add water and groats to rice bowl and let soak overnight or during the day. When ready to cook, add an additional 1 cup of water and turn machine on. Let grain steam for 10 additional minutes after it has turned off. If you have not soaked them, your cooking time will be closer to 90 minutes.

Serves 4

Nutrition Facts

Serving Size 1.675 ounces (47.50g)
Servings Per Container 4

Amount Per Serving

Calories 171   Calories from Fat 12

	% Daily Value*
Total Fat 1g	2%
Saturated Fat 0g	0%
Cholesterol 0mg	0%
Sodium 2mg	0%
Total Carbohydrate 32g	11%
Dietary Fiber 1g	4%
Sugars 0g	
Protein 8g	

Vitamin A -%	Vitamin C -%
Calcium 1%	Iron -%

*Percent Daily Values are based on a 2,000 calorie diet. Your daily values may be higher or lower depending on your calorie needs.

Breakfast Kamut

For a quick start, let the grains soak overnight.

1 cup Kamut, presoaked
1 cup lowfat milk or soy milk
½ cup sultana raisins
1 tablespoon honey
Salt to taste

Plastic Steamers
Fill water reservoir to maximum and turn on machine. Add drained Kamut, milk, and sultanas to rice bowl and steam for 50 minutes. Drizzle Kamut with honey before serving.

Metal Steamers
Coat rice bowl with nonstick spray. Add drained Kamut, milk, sultanas, and an additional 1 cup of water to rice bowl. Turn on machine. Let Kamut steam for 10 additional minutes after steamer switches to warm. Drizzle with honey before serving.

Serves 4

Nutrition Facts	
Serving Size 4.762 ounces (135.0g)	
Servings Per Container 4	
Amount Per Serving	
Calories 276 Calories from Fat 18	
	% *Daily Value**
Total Fat 2g	3%
Saturated Fat 1g	5%
Cholesterol 2mg	1%
Sodium 35mg	1%
Total Carbohydrate 56g	19%
Dietary Fiber 2g	8%
Sugars 7g	
Protein 11g	
Vitamin A 3%	Vitamin C 2%
Calcium 10%	Iron 2%

*Percent Daily Values are based on a 2,000 calorie diet. Your daily values may be higher or lower depending on your calorie needs.

Kamut Pilaf with Currants and Cumin

The rich cumin flavor along with the tang of currants make this a special little recipe.

2 cups lowfat chicken broth
1 cup Kamut groats, presoaked
3 tablespoons fresh parsley, chopped
2 tablespoons currants
1 teaspoon cumin seeds

Plastic Steamers

Fill water reservoir to maximum and turn on steamer. Add ingredients and steam for 50 to 60 minutes until grain is soft and chewy. If grain is not cooked when machine turns off, add more water to reservoir and rice bowl, if needed.

Metal Steamers

Coat rice bowl with nonstick spray. Add ingredients with an additional 1 cup of water. Let grain steam for 10 additional minutes on warm after machine turns off.

Serves 4

Nutrition Facts	
Serving Size 5.959 ounces (168.9g)	
Servings Per Container 4	
Amount Per Serving	
Calories 198 Calories from Fat 18	
	% *Daily Value**
Total Fat 2g	3%
Saturated Fat 0g	0%
Cholesterol 0mg	0%
Sodium 172mg	7%
Total Carbohydrate 37g	12%
Dietary Fiber 1g	4%
Sugars 0g	
Protein 11g	
Vitamin A 1%	Vitamin C 4%
Calcium 2%	Iron 4%

*Percent Daily Values are based on a 2,000 calorie diet. Your daily values may be higher or lower depending on your calorie needs.

Daniella's Three Grain Salad

This salad has an unusual texture and a refreshing flavor. One of our favorite grain salads.

1 cup cooked Kamut
1 cup cooked barley
1 cup cooked rice
¼ cup finely chopped fresh mint
¼ cup chopped dried cranberries
2 tablespoons balsamic vinegar
Salt to taste

Combine ingredients, chill, and serve.

Serves 4

Nutrition Facts	
Serving Size 3.571 ounces (101.2g)	
Servings Per Container 4	

Amount Per Serving

Calories 275   Calories from Fat 15

	% Daily Value*
Total Fat 2g	3%
Saturated Fat 0g	0%
Cholesterol 0mg	0%
Sodium 6mg	0%
Total Carbohydrate 57g	19%
Dietary Fiber 2g	8%
Sugars 0g	
Protein 8g	

Vitamin A 4%	Vitamin C 20%
Calcium 3%	Iron 10%

*Percent Daily Values are based on a 2,000 calorie diet. Your daily values may be higher or lower depending on your calorie needs.

Kamut and Creamy Rice Farina

This porridge has a delightful mouth feel and light, sweet flavor.

3 cups water
¾ cup creamy rice farina
¼ cup Kamut flour
2 tablespoons sunflower seeds
2 tablespoons honey or other sweetener
1 tablespoon amaranth seeds, lightly toasted
Salt to taste

Plastic Steamers

Fill water reservoir to maximum and turn on steamer. Add ingredients and steam for 60 to 70 minutes until grain is soft and chewy. If grain is not cooked when machine turns off, add more water to reservoir and rice bowl, if needed.

Metal Steamers

Coat rice bowl with nonstick spray. Add ingredients with an additional 1 cup of water. Let grain steam for 10 additional minutes on warm after machine turns off.

Serves 4

Nutrition Facts

Serving Size 1.973 ounces (55.94g)
Servings Per Container 4

Amount Per Serving

Calories 207   Calories from Fat 23

	% Daily Value*
Total Fat 3g	5%
Saturated Fat 0g	0%
Cholesterol 0mg	0%
Sodium 2mg	0%
Total Carbohydrate 40g	13%
Dietary Fiber 2g	8%
Sugars 9g	
Protein 6g	

Vitamin A 0%	Vitamin C 0%
Calcium 1%	Iron 8%

*Percent Daily Values are based on a 2,000 calorie diet. Your daily values may be higher or lower depending on your calorie needs.

Kamut Olé

This spicy old number has a new twist, and it's for the better.
Try this as an alternative to vegetarian chili.

1 cup water
1 cup Kamut, presoaked
8-ounce can peeled whole tomatoes
½ cup green onions, sliced
½ cup finely chopped celery
1 teaspoon cumin powder
½ teaspoon chili powder
1 clove chopped garlic (or 1 teaspoon powder)
1 can adzuki beans

Plastic Steamers
Add maximum amount of water
to reservoir and turn on machine. Place all ingredients except beans and tomatoes in rice
bowl and steam for 60 minutes.
When grains are tender, add
beans and tomatoes and warm
them for 5 additional minutes.

Metal Steamer
Coat bottom of rice bowl with a
nonstick spray. Add all ingredients except beans and tomatoes
plus 1 cup of water to the rice
bowl and cook for 60 minutes.
When steamer switches to
warm, add beans and tomatoes
and steam on warm for 10 minutes.

Nutrition Facts	
Serving Size 6.507 ounces (184.5g)	
Servings Per Container 4	
Amount Per Serving	
Calories 267 Calories from Fat 15	
	% *Daily Value**
Total Fat 2g	3%
Saturated Fat 0g	0%
Cholesterol 0mg	0%
Sodium 184mg	8%
Total Carbohydrate 52g	17%
Dietary Fiber 5g	20%
Sugars 0g	
Protein 13g	
Vitamin A 5%	Vitamin C 17%
Calcium 6%	Iron 11%

*Percent Daily Values are based on a
2,000 calorie diet. Your daily values
may be higher or lower depending on
your calorie needs.

Serves 4

Ancient Grain Salad

This is a combination of several ancient grains. To make cold grain salads quickly, cook a large quantity of your favorite grains and store them in the refrigerator for up to a week. This salad will serve as a lunch or dinner during hot weather.

This recipe also works well with wheat berries, oat groats, and brown rice.

1 cup cooked Kamut, cooled
1 cup cooked spelt, cooled
1 cup cooked quinoa, cooled
1 cup parsley, finely chopped
1½ cups (about 1 pound) large, cooked shrimp
½ cup green onion, chopped
3 tablespoons fresh mint, chopped

Dressing

½ cup lime juice
4 tablespoons virgin olive oil
½ teaspoon dried oregano
½ teaspoon dried ground cumin
¼ teaspoon freshly ground
   black pepper

Combine ingredients and fluff with fork. Toss with dressing and chill in refrigerator to mingle flavors. Serve cold.

Serves 6 as a side dish, 3 as a main course

Nutrition Facts	
Serving Size 5.947 ounces (168.6g)	
Servings Per Container 6	
Amount Per Serving	
Calories 303 Calories from Fat 99	
	% *Daily Value**
Total Fat 11g	17%
Saturated Fat 2g	10%
Cholesterol 114mg	38%
Sodium 574mg	24%
Total Carbohydrate 31g	10%
Dietary Fiber 2g	8%
Sugars 1g	
Protein 22g	
Vitamin A 15%	Vitamin C 41%
Calcium 11%	Iron 17%

*Percent Daily Values are based on a 2,000 calorie diet. Your daily values may be higher or lower depending on your calorie needs.

Kamut with Apple and Celery

This salad is very simple to make but delicious. If you do not have any cooked Kamut on hand, substitute barley groats, oat groats, brown rice, wheat berries, rye berries, or spelt.

2 cups cooked Kamut, cooled
1 cup lowfat cottage cheese
½ cup chopped red apple
½ cup chopped celery
¼ cup finely chopped onion
4 cups shredded butter lettuce

Combine Kamut, cottage cheese, apple, celery, and onion. Arrange 1 cup of lettuce on each salad plate and place 1 cup of Kamut mixture onto lettuce.

Serves 4

Nutrition Facts	
Serving Size 5.273 ounces (149.5g)	
Servings Per Container 6	
Amount Per Serving	
Calories 158 Calories from Fat 13	
	% *Daily Value**
Total Fat 1g	2%
Saturated Fat 0g	0%
Cholesterol 2mg	1%
Sodium 166mg	7%
Total Carbohydrate 26g	9%
Dietary Fiber 2g	8%
Sugars 3g	
Protein 11g	
Vitamin A 5%	Vitamin C 9%
Calcium 5%	Iron 1%

*Percent Daily Values are based on a 2,000 calorie diet. Your daily values may be higher or lower depending on your calorie needs.

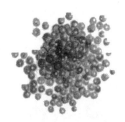

CHAPTER 10

Millet (*Panicum miliaceum*)

This small, yellow, beadlike grain has a mild, nutty flavor and fluffy texture.

Millets are natives of Africa or Asia and have been cultivated for over six thousand years. The earliest documents that mention millet were found in China and date back to about 2800 B.C. They refer to the grain as a "holy plant." The Bible calls millet "the gruel of endurance." It was once the staple grain of India, Egypt, and North Africa. During the medieval era, millet was one of the principal grains of Europe and the people of Java reportedly grew millet around their rice fields to activate growth of the rice plant and encourage abundance.

What Is Millet?

Millet is the small, round seed of an annual grass that is eaten as a cereal in Africa and Asia. Millet is not a true cereal grain but is instead related to sorghum, a type of millet that is the staple food of the Hunzas, the Himalayan tribespeople known for their longevity. This grain is important in arid countries because it will grow with very little water and poor soil.

Steamed millet has a light, delicate flavor with an ideal texture for molding. Pan-roasted millet tastes like toasted cashew nuts.

Nutrition and Millet

Millet is a good source of protein and contains more of the limiting amino acid, lysine, than do wheat, oats, and rice. One cup of millet provides almost 20% of the day's protein requirement. Millet is also an excellent source of the B vitamins thiamin, riboflavin, niacin, pyridoxine, and folate and of the minerals magnesium, zinc, copper, and iron.

Because millet is also a rich source of the mineral-binding phytochemical phytic acid, you should always include a vitamin C–rich food in the same meal with which millet is served. Sources of vitamin C are listed in chapter 5.

Health and Millet

Esophageal Cancer

Populations where millet is a staple have a lower risk of developing esophageal cancer that those where wheat and corn are the staple foods. This may be due to the high concentrations of magnesium, zinc, riboflavin, and nicotinic acid in millet.

Cancer Prevention

Millet is rich in phytate. This phytochemical appears to reduce colon and mammary gland cancer risk in animals.

How to Buy Millet

Millet can usually be purchased only as a whole grain. You will find it in some supermarkets but will probably have to go to a health food store to find it. Millet is sold in boxes and out of bins for bulk buying. Millet sold as bird seed has not been de-hulled. Unless you have a beak, buy millet sold only for human consumption!

Look for grains that are bright gold in color. The dark grains are seeds that escaped hulling. Millet normally has little or no odor. If you detect a musty smell, do not buy it.

Millet has a long shelf life. Like all grains, it should be kept in a sealed container and stored in a dark, cool place. Raw millet can be stored for up to six months. Cooked millet can be stored for up to three days in the refrigerator.

How to Use Millet

Millet is an extremely versatile grain. It can be steamed di-rectly or toasted in a dry skillet before steaming. Cooked mil-let makes an excellent porridge or pudding. It can also be served as a pilaf, a stuffing, or an addition to soups and green salads. Raw, it can be added to other grains as a crunchy top-ping. Raw millet is a smart alternative to fat-rich nuts and seeds.

Recipes

Basic Cooking Instructions

Millet readily absorbs water, so be prepared to add extra. This grain has a light, delicate flavor that takes on the character of whatever it is cooked with. Be creative in your choice of cook-ing liquids.

1 cup millet, toasted or plain
1 cup water, juice, or broth
Salt to taste

Plastic Steamers

Fill water reservoir and turn on machine. Add ingredients to rice bowl and steam for 35 to 45 minutes.

Metal Steamers

Coat rice bowl with nonstick spray. Add millet and cooking liquid to rice bowl with an additional 1 cup of water. Turn on machine and cook until machine turns off. Stir grains, season to taste, and let steam for an additional 5 minutes.

Toasted Millet

Place raw grain in a hot, dry skillet and stir until grains turn a slight golden brown. Be careful not to overcook. Toasted millet can be stored for up to two days in the refrigerator before steaming, but it is better if steamed immediately.

Serves 4

Nutrition Facts

Serving Size 1.764 ounces (50.00g)
Servings Per Container 4

Amount Per Serving

Calories 189   Calories from Fat 19

	% Daily Value*
Total Fat 2g	3%
Saturated Fat 0g	0%
Cholesterol 0mg	0%
Sodium 2mg	0%
Total Carbohydrate 36g	12%
Dietary Fiber 7g	28%
Sugars 0g	
Protein 6g	

Vitamin A 0%	Vitamin C 0%
Calcium 0%	Iron 8%

*Percent Daily Values are based on a 2,000 calorie diet. Your daily values may be higher or lower depending on your calorie needs.

Breakfast Millet

Millet really picks up the flavor of the sweetener, so vary the sweetener to vary the taste. We really love molasses—the flavor and color that it adds to this cereal.

1¼ cups milk
1 cup water
¾ cup millet
2 tablespoons liquid sweetener
Salt to taste

Optional: Sprinkle top with seeds or nuts, serve in a bowl of milk, drizzle with honey or maple syrup.

Plastic Steamers
Fill water reservoir and turn on machine. Add ingredients to rice bowl and steam for 40 minutes.

Metal Steamers
Coat rice bowl with nonstick spray. Add millet and cooking liquid to rice bowl with an additional 1 cup of water. Turn on machine and cook until machine turns off. Stir grains, season to taste, and let steam for an additional 5 minutes.

Serves 4

Nutrition Facts	
Serving Size 4.374 ounces (124.0g)	
Servings Per Container 4	
Amount Per Serving	
Calories 195 Calories from Fat 22	
	% *Daily Value**
Total Fat 2g	3%
Saturated Fat 1g	5%
Cholesterol 3mg	1%
Sodium 50mg	2%
Total Carbohydrate 37g	12%
Dietary Fiber 5g	20%
Sugars 3g	
Protein 7g	
Vitamin A 4%	Vitamin C 1%
Calcium 16%	Iron 15%

*Percent Daily Values are based on a 2,000 calorie diet. Your daily values may be higher or lower depending on your calorie needs.

Millet Pilaf

This flavorful dish can be modified to include your favorite vegetables. Red peppers and celery are refreshing additions.

1 cup millet
1 can vegetable broth
1 cup chopped parsley
1 tomato, chopped
½ cup chopped green onion
Salt and pepper to taste

Plastic Steamers

Fill water reservoir and turn on machine. Add ingredients to rice bowl and steam for 35 to 45 minutes.

Metal Steamers

Coat rice bowl with nonstick spray. Add millet and cooking liquid to rice bowl with an additional 1 cup of water. Turn on machine and cook until machine turns off. Stir grains, season to taste, and let steam for an additional 5 minutes.

Serves 4

Nutrition Facts	
Serving Size 5.586 ounces (158.4g)	
Servings Per Container 4	
Amount Per Serving	
Calories 211 Calories from Fat 24	
	% *Daily Value**
Total Fat 3g	5%
Saturated Fat 0g	0%
Cholesterol 0mg	0%
Sodium 206mg	9%
Total Carbohydrate 39g	13%
Dietary Fiber 8g	32%
Sugars 1g	
Protein 7g	
Vitamin A 10%	Vitamin C 34%
Calcium 2%	Iron 15%

*Percent Daily Values are based on a 2,000 calorie diet. Your daily values may be higher or lower depending on your calorie needs.

Millet and Potato

A pleasant change from mashed potatoes.

2 tablespoons vegetable oil
½ teaspoon mustard seeds
1½ cups cooked millet
1 medium potato, well-scrubbed
1 teaspoon chopped, fresh ginger or ⅛ teaspoon dry ginger
    powder
Salt to taste
½ teaspoon curry powder

Heat oil in medium frying pan and add mustard seeds. When the mustard seeds pop, add them to millet. Wash and dice potato and add to millet. Add ginger, salt, and curry powder.

Serves 4

Nutrition Facts	
Serving Size 4.644 ounces (131.7g)	
Servings Per Container 4	
Amount Per Serving	
Calories 199 Calories from Fat 71	
	% *Daily Value**
Total Fat 8g	12%
Saturated Fat 1g	5%
Cholesterol 0mg	0%
Sodium 4mg	0%
Total Carbohydrate 28g	9%
Dietary Fiber 5g	20%
Sugars 1g	
Protein 4g	
Vitamin A 0%	Vitamin C 4%
Calcium 0%	Iron 4%

*Percent Daily Values are based on a 2,000 calorie diet. Your daily values may be higher or lower depending on your calorie needs.

Millet Salad

As good tasting as it is good looking. This salad can also double as a stuffing.

1 cup lowfat chicken or vegetable broth
⅔ cup water
½ cup millet
½ cup dried apricots, chopped
½ cup carrot, grated
¼ cup toasted almonds, chopped
¼ cup green onions, chopped
¼ teaspoon saffron

Plastic Steamers
Fill water reservoir and turn on machine. Add ingredients to rice bowl and steam for 20 minutes. Place into ½-cup molds and serve on a bed of spinach.

Metal Steamers
Coat rice bowl with nonstick spray. Add ingredients to rice bowl with an additional ½ cup of water. Turn on machine and cook until machine turns off. Place into ½-cup molds and serve on a bed of spinach.

Serves 4

Nutrition Facts	
Serving Size 4.239 ounces (120.2g)	
Servings Per Container 4	

Amount Per Serving	
Calories 188 Calories from Fat 47	

	% *Daily Value**
Total Fat 5g	8%
Saturated Fat 1g	5%
Cholesterol 0mg	0%
Sodium 92mg	4%
Total Carbohydrate 32g	11%
Dietary Fiber 6g	24%
Sugars 8g	
Protein 6g	

Vitamin A 51%	Vitamin C 3%
Calcium 3%	Iron 11%

*Percent Daily Values are based on a 2,000 calorie diet. Your daily values may be higher or lower depending on your calorie needs.

Herbed Millet

This simple spicy dish really jazzes up a dinner.

1 cup millet
2½ to 3 cups vegetable broth
½ small onion, finely chopped
3 small cloves garlic, unpeeled (or 1 peeled and minced)
1 teaspoon sage

Plastic Steamers
Fill water reservoir and turn on machine. Add ingredients to rice bowl and steam for 40 minutes.

Metal Steamers
Coat rice bowl with nonstick spray. Add ingredients to rice bowl with an additional 1 cup of water. Turn on machine and cook until machine turns off.

Serves 6

Nutrition Facts	
Serving Size 1.468 ounces (41.62g)	
Servings Per Container 6	
Amount Per Serving	
Calories 131 Calories from Fat 13	
	% *Daily Value**
Total Fat 1g	2%
Saturated Fat 0g	0%
Cholesterol 0mg	0%
Sodium 2mg	0%
Total Carbohydrate 25g	8%
Dietary Fiber 5g	20%
Sugars 0g	
Protein 4g	
Vitamin A 0%	Vitamin C 1%
Calcium 0%	Iron 5%

*Percent Daily Values are based on a 2,000 calorie diet. Your daily values may be higher or lower depending on your calorie needs.

Millet Burgers

Millet has a wonderful texture for shaping into patties. We like to grill these burgers outside on our grill.

4 cups cooked millet (made with broth)
2 lightly beaten eggs
½ cup wheat germ
2 tablespoons nutritional yeast
2 garlic cloves, crushed
2 tablespoons low-salt soy sauce
2 tablespoons catsup
whole wheat flour or corn flour

Divide and form the mixture into 6 patties of approximately equal size. Dust patties with flour. Place on preheated pan to which 1 tablespoon of olive oil has been added. Lightly fry patties on both sides and serve with tomato and lettuce on a whole wheat bun.

To freeze uncooked patties, separate each patty with wax paper and store in freezer bag.

Serves 6

Nutrition Facts	
Serving Size 6.863 ounces (194.6g)	
Servings Per Container 6	

Amount Per Serving	
Calories 244 Calories from Fat 34	

	% *Daily Value**
Total Fat 4g	6%
Saturated Fat 1g	5%
Cholesterol 71mg	24%
Sodium 270mg	9%
Total Carbohydrate 43g	14%
Dietary Fiber 9g	36%
Sugars 1g	
Protein 10g	

Vitamin A 3%	Vitamin C 1%
Calcium 3%	Iron 11%

*Percent Daily Values are based on a 2,000 calorie diet. Your daily values may be higher or lower depending on your calorie needs.

CHAPTER 11

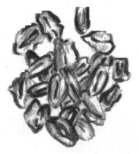

Oats (*Avena sativa*)

The whole grains, or groats, are rolled to produce the familiar flakes used for porridge.

Oats originated in Europe or Asia. The first evidence of the use of oats was found at the Franchthi Cave in Greece at a level dated to 10,500 B.C. The oat plant used to be considered a weed and was used only for medical purposes. Theophrastus and Pliny actually considered oats to be a diseased form of wheat.

What Are Oats?

Oats are a true cereal grain; but compared to other true cereals, they have a higher protein and fat content. The physical structure of the oat kernel is similar to that of the kernels of wheat and barley. The oat seed or groat is contained within a hull which must be removed before the seed can be eaten. This makes oats difficult to process, since the oat husk is very adherent.

When oats are dehulled, the bran and germ remain with the groat. This is what makes oats such an excellent source of B vitamins and minerals.

Oats contain gluten which makes them unsuitable for individuals with celiac disease.

Nutrition and Oats

Oats are a good source of protein. One cup of cooked oat groats will supply an adult with 29% of the protein they need for a day. Oats are also rich in the B-complex vitamins thiamin, folate, and pantothenic acid; the minerals iron, magnesium, copper, and zinc. Oats are also a source of linoleic acid, an essential fatty acid. Oats additionally are famous for their fiber content. Oat bran is so rich in soluble fiber, it has become synonymous with low cholesterol.

Health and Oats

Before 1988, oat bran was a specialty item that was available only through health food stores. Then, in April of 1988, a paper concerning oat bran appeared in the *Journal of the American Medical Association*. The article concluded that oat bran could be used as an alternative to drugs for some individuals with high serum cholesterol. When the article was picked up by the media, oat bran sales exploded and soon even the entire oat milling industry was depleted of oat bran. Product had to be imported from Europe to meet the demand.

Can Oats Reduce High Cholesterol?

A number of studies performed since 1988 have confirmed oats' ability to reduce the serum-cholesterol levels. Oat bran does not lower the cholesterol of people with normal levels, only of those with high levels. How oat bran accomplishes this reduction in cholesterol is not yet known, but it is likely due to a combination of factors rather than just one. Some of the reasons oats can reduce cholesterol are listed below.

- Insulin increases cholesterol synthesis; soluble fibers reduce after-meal hyperglycemia and associated insulin elevations, which may reduce cholesterol synthesis.
- Oats also contain alpha tocotrienol, a form of vitamin E, which may lower cholesterol.
- Propionate and acetate, two of the short chain fatty acids produced in the colon from soluble fiber, are believed to be responsible for some of the hypocholesteremic properties of oats. These products are absorbed into the blood and make their way to the liver, the site of cholesterol synthesis. In the liver they inhibit the production of cholesterol.
- Cholesterol is a component of the bile secreted to emulsify fats in the intestine. Soluble fiber may reduce the reabsorption of cholesterol from the bile acids in the small intestine.
- Beta-glucan, a gum that is found in the endosperm of the groat, is believed to lower cholesterol.
- Two saponins found in oats, avenacoside A and B, have been implicated in oats' ability to reduce cholesterol. These saponins have been shown to bind to cholesterol in the test tube. In the intestine, they may do the same and bind cholesterol so that it cannot be absorbed and is excreted from the body. The amount of avenacosides appears to decrease with the amount of processing. Again, it is best to eat your grain as unprocessed as possible.

Hypoglycemia and Diabetes

The soluble fiber in oats decreases the rate at which the stomach empties, therefore moderating the amount of sugar available to the blood. This keeps blood sugar levels even and avoids the dips in sugar that trigger insulin release.

Osteoporosis

Oats are a good source of manganese, which is important for bone metabolism. Researchers have found that animals who are deficient in this trace mineral are at risk for developing severe osteoporosis.

Menopausal Symptoms

Oats are a good source of phytoestrogens—plant estrogens. Plant estrogens appear to be able to alleviate symptoms of menopause without cancer-promoting effects.

Cancer Prevention

Oats are good sources of cancer-preventing antioxidants. Oat powder is even used commercially to coat foods to prevent oxidative damage and reduce spoilage.

Immune Functioning

The saponins found in oats have some antibiotic properties.

How to Buy Oats

Oats can be purchased in sealed packages or from bulk bins. We like to purchase oats in bulk from bins, because it enables us to buy as much or as little as we want. If allergies are a concern, however, avoid buying from bins because there may be cross-contamination between bins. You may end up with more than you thought you bought.

Oats have many different uses, and many different kinds of oats are available.

Oat Groats

Oat groats are the entire oat kernel minus only the hull. It contains all of the germ and bran.

Steel-Cut Oats

Steel-cut oats are made by passing whole groats through steel cutting machines. These oats contain all of the bran and germ and make a chewy, hearty porridge.

Scotch-Cut Oats

Scotch-cut oats are made by grinding groats with stones. The result is a fine grind of oats which makes a very creamy porridge.

Rolled Oats

Rolled oats are made by slicing steamed groats and rolling the pieces into flakes. Rolled oats are available as thick or medium flakes and require less cooking time than steel-cut oats or whole oat groats.

Quick Oats

Quick oats are made from very thin slices of groats that are passed over a heat source during rolling, which partially cooks them. Quick oats cook faster than rolled oats but have less texture.

Instant Oats

Instant oats are made from very thin slices of groats which are rolled and then precooked. They are the most processed form of oats available. Only boiling water is needed to produce a cooked hot cereal. Instant oats have very little texture and should not be used in breads or other baked goods.

Oat Bran

Oat bran is a purified product that contains only the soluble fiber–rich bran layer. It makes a hearty hot cereal, or it can be added to other grains to increase the soluble fiber content.

How to Use Oats

Rolled oats can be used for breakfast cereals, and oat groats and steel-cut oats make excellent substitutes for rice in pilafs and stuffings. Oat bran is a well-known supplement that can be added to a variety of grain dishes.

Since oats are very high in unsaturated fatty acids, you might suspect that they would have special storage requirements. However, a natural antioxidant protects the fats in oats from becoming rancid. Oats can be stored for up to one year in a cool, dry place.

Recipes

Basic Cooking Instructions

These instructions can be used to cook any rolled grain, including rolled barley, triticale, spelt, and wheat. Rolled cereals make quick and tasty breakfast cereals. Serve this recipe with milk and honey drizzled on top.

1 cup rolled oats
1 cup water, juice, or milk
1 tablespoon date sugar or Succanet
Salt to taste

Plastic Steamers
Fill reservoir to minimum level and turn on machine. Add ingredients and steam for 15 minutes.

Metal Steamers
Coat rice bowl with nonstick spray. Add ingredients and turn on machine. Cook until machine turns off. Serve immediately.

Serves 4

Nutrition Facts

Serving Size 0.714 ounces (20.25g)
Servings Per Container 4

Amount Per Serving

Calories 78   Calories from Fat 11

	% *Daily Value**
Total Fat 1g	2%
Saturated Fat 0g	0%
Cholesterol 0mg	0%
Sodium 1mg	0%
Total Carbohydrate 14g	5%
Dietary Fiber 1g	4%
Sugars 0g	
Protein 3g	

Vitamin A 0%	Vitamin C 0%
Calcium 1%	Iron 4%

---

*Percent Daily Values are based on a 2,000 calorie diet. Your daily values may be higher or lower depending on your calorie needs.

Maureen's Breakfast Oatmeal

The very best oatmeal we have ever tasted. There is simply no better way to start your day. The date sugar adds a not-too-sweet crunchy topping that contrasts nicely with the creamy oatmeal.

1 cup scotch-cut oats
1 cup water
1 tablespoon date sugar (crushed dates)
1 teaspoon salt
8 dried apple rings
4 tablespoons date sugar (topping)
1 cup 1% fat milk

Plastic Steamers

Fill reservoir to minimum with water and turn on machine. Add oats, water, 1 tablespoon date sugar, and salt to rice bowl. Lay apple rings on top of ingredients. Steam for 15 to 20 minutes. Then see below.

Metal Steamers

Coat rice bowl with nonstick spray. Add oats, water, 1 tablespoon date sugar, and salt to machine. Lay apple rings on top of ingredients. Cook until machine turns off and let steam for 5 minutes on warm.

Nutrition Facts	
Serving Size 3.784 ounces (107.3g)	
Servings Per Container 4	
Amount Per Serving	
Calories 168 Calories from Fat 18	
	% *Daily Value**
Total Fat 2g	3%
Saturated Fat 1g	5%
Cholesterol 2mg	1%
Sodium 574mg	24%
Total Carbohydrate 34g	11%
Dietary Fiber 3g	12%
Sugars 12g	
Protein 6g	
Vitamin A 4%	Vitamin C 1%
Calcium 9%	Iron 6%

*Percent Daily Values are based on a 2,000 calorie diet. Your daily values may be higher or lower depending on your calorie needs.

Lay two apple rings in center of each of four bowls and place half cup of oatmeal on top of apples. We like to use a 4-ounce (½ cup) measuring cup as a mold. Pour ¼ cup of milk around oatmeal and carefully spoon 1 tablespoon date sugar on top.

Serves 4

Granola Oatmeal

You can substitute any cereal you have on hand for the granola. Vanilla soy milk works especially well here. There are many variations possible; have fun with it.

¾ cup thick rolled oats
½ cup granola
1¼ cups water
Salt to taste
Honey, soy milk, almond milk, or dairy milk (optional)

Plastic Steamers

Fill reservoir with minimum amount of water and turn on machine. Add ingredients and steam for 20 minutes. Then see below.

Metal Steamers

Coat rice bowl with nonstick spray and add ingredients. Cook for 15 minutes and steam on warm for an additional 5 minutes.

Serve oatmeal with a moat of milk. Garnish by sprinkling a little granola on top of each bowl. Drizzle a little honey or maple syrup on top for a sweeter treat.

Serves 4

Nutrition Facts	
Serving Size 1.034 ounces (29.31g)	
Servings Per Container 4	
Amount Per Serving	
Calories 121 Calories from Fat 31	
	% *Daily Value**
Total Fat 3g	5%
Saturated Fat 2g	10%
Cholesterol 0mg	0%
Sodium 30mg	1%
Total Carbohydrate 20g	7%
Dietary Fiber 1g	4%
Sugars 4g	
Protein 4g	
Vitamin A 0%	Vitamin C 0%
Calcium 1%	Iron 6%

*Percent Daily Values are based on a 2,000 calorie diet. Your daily values may be higher or lower depending on your calorie needs.

Toasted Oat Pilaf

A delicious change from rice.

1½ cups toasted oat groats
1½ cups fresh or canned tomato juice
1 tablespoon chopped fresh rosemary
Pepper to taste
1 tablespoon fresh chopped cilantro

Plastic Steamers

Add oats and tomato juice to rice bowl and let soak for 6 to 8 hours (or overnight). Fill reservoir to maximum with water and turn on machine. Add rosemary and pepper. Steam for 60 minutes. Add cilantro and serve.

Metal Steamers

Coat rice bowl with nonstick spray and add toasted oats and tomato juice. Let soak for 6 to 8 hours (or overnight). Add rosemary, pepper, and 1 cup water. Cook until machine turns off and then let steam for 10 minutes on warm. Add cilantro and serve.

Serves 6

Nutrition Facts	
Serving Size 3.554 ounces (100.8g)	
Servings Per Container 6	
Amount Per Serving	
Calories 163 Calories from Fat 25	
	% *Daily Value**
Total Fat 3g	5%
Saturated Fat 0g	0%
Cholesterol 0mg	0%
Sodium 7mg	0%
Total Carbohydrate 29g	10%
Dietary Fiber 6g	24%
Sugars 3g	
Protein 7g	
Vitamin A 3%	Vitamin C 19%
Calcium 2%	Iron 12%

*Percent Daily Values are based on a 2,000 calorie diet. Your daily values may be higher or lower depending on your calorie needs.

Oat Salad

Try this as an alternative to potato salad. It's a heart-healthy choice.

1 cup steel-cut oats
1 cup lowfat chicken broth
½ cup chopped water chestnuts
½ teaspoon turmeric
1 tablespoon gourmet mustard
1 tablespoon mayonnaise
1 green onion, chopped
Paprika for garnish

Plastic Steamers
Fill reservoir with maximum amount of water and turn on machine. Add oats, broth, water chestnuts, and turmeric to rice bowl and steam for 40 minutes. Cool and add mustard, mayonnaise, and green onion. Scoop onto a bed of lettuce. Sprinkle with paprika.

Metal Steamers
Coat rice bowl with nonstick spray and add oats, broth, water chestnuts, turmeric, and an additional ⅔ cup water. When machine turns off, steam on warm for an additional 5 minutes. Cool and add mustard, mayonnaise, and green onion. Scoop onto a bed of lettuce. Sprinkle with paprika.

Serves 4

Nutrition Facts	
Serving Size 4.467 ounces (126.6g)	
Servings Per Container 4	

Amount Per Serving	
Calories 201 Calories from Fat 55	

	% Daily Value*
Total Fat 6g	9%
Saturated Fat 1g	5%
Cholesterol 2mg	1%
Sodium 266mg	11%
Total Carbohydrate 29g	10%
Dietary Fiber 5g	20%
Sugars 1g	
Protein 8g	

Vitamin A 0%	Vitamin C 1%
Calcium 3%	Iron 13%

*Percent Daily Values are based on a 2,000 calorie diet. Your daily values may be higher or lower depending on your calorie needs.

Oat Pudding

This comfort food is wonderful warm and with a drizzle of maple syrup on top.

1 cup scotch-cut oats
1½ cups vanilla soy milk
¼ cup raisins or dates, chopped finely
1 tablespoon date sugar or Succanet
1 teaspoon cinnamon
1 teaspoon nutmeg
Salt to taste

Plastic Steamers
Fill reservoir to minimum level and turn on machine. Add ingredients and steam for 15 minutes. Serve.

Metal Steamers
Coat rice bowl with nonstick spray. Add ingredients and turn on machine. Cook until machine turns off. Serve immediately.

Serves 4

Nutrition Facts	
Serving Size 5.116 ounces (145.0g)	
Servings Per Container 4	

Amount Per Serving	
Calories 252 Calories from Fat 44	

	% *Daily Value**
Total Fat 5g	8%
Saturated Fat 1g	5%
Cholesterol 0mg	0%
Sodium 47mg	2%
Total Carbohydrate 45g	15%
Dietary Fiber 6g	24%
Sugars 2g	
Protein 9g	

Vitamin A 18%	Vitamin C 1%
Calcium 14%	Iron 16%

*Percent Daily Values are based on a 2,000 calorie diet. Your daily values may be higher or lower depending on your calorie needs.

Apple and Oat Breakfast

A high fiber start to the morning. The apple juice gives this recipe a fragrant light sweetness.

1 cup steel-cut oats
1½ cups apple juice
1 teaspoon apple pie spice
1 tablespoon flaxseeds or psyllium seed
1 tablespoon sunflower seeds
1 tablespoon rice polish or bran

Plastic Steamers
Fill reservoir to maximum level and turn on machine. Add ingredients and steam for 40 minutes. Serve.

Metal Steamers
Coat rice bowl with nonstick spray. Add ingredients plus an additional ⅓ to ½ cup of water and turn on machine. Cook until machine turns off. Serve immediately.

Serves 4

Nutrition Facts	
Serving Size 4.933 ounces (139.9g)	
Servings Per Container 4	
Amount Per Serving	
Calories 232 Calories from Fat 48	
	% *Daily Value**
Total Fat 5g	8%
Saturated Fat 1g	5%
Cholesterol 0mg	0%
Sodium 6mg	0%
Total Carbohydrate 40g	13%
Dietary Fiber 6g	24%
Sugars 11g	
Protein 8g	
Vitamin A 0%	Vitamin C 1%
Calcium 4%	Iron 17%
*Percent Daily Values are based on a 2,000 calorie diet. Your daily values may be higher or lower depending on your calorie needs.	

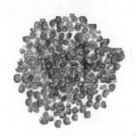

Quinoa (Chenopodium quinoa)

This small, disk-shaped seed is light beige and has a delicate, fluffy texture.

Quinoa originated in the Andean region of South America. The importance of quinoa to the Incas is demonstrated by the name the Quechua gave it, "chisiya mama," which means "mother grain." Francisco Pizarro is said to have made the comment that quinoa is "the grain that grows where grass will not." The cultivation of quinoa was discouraged after the conquest because of its importance in Inca society and religion. In Columbia, the cultivation of quinoa was abandoned almost entirely; and in Ecuador, Bolivia, Chile, and Argentina, only enough was grown to feed the local peasants. This led to quinoa's being stigmatized as a poor person's food.

Quinoa was reintroduced to the States in 1982 and has become increasingly popular at health food stores.

What Is Quinoa?

Quinoa, pronounced *keen-wa*, is not a true cereal but a pseudocereal. It belongs to the *Chenopodium*, or goosefoot, family and so is related to spinach. Quinoa is frost-resistant and able to grow in poor soils with low rainfall. The seeds are round and flattened, with a small bran band around the middle. They are so small it takes 350 grains to weigh 1 gram. The grain becomes transparent when cooked, and the bran layer becomes visible as a curly tail.

Quinoa seeds are coated with saponins, a bitter compound that may act as a built-in pest deterrent. They are washed and scrubbed to remove these bitter but harmless compounds before packaging. Package directions recommend a second washing at home before cooking.

Nutrition and Quinoa

Quinoa's claim to fame is its amino acid content. It is very rich in protein. The National Academy of Sciences has called quinoa the best source of protein in the vegetable kingdom. It is higher in protein than the true cereal grains. What's more, the protein is of high quality, since the grain is rich in histadine and lysine—two amino acids that are usually limited in grains—and high in methionine and cysteine, two amino acids limited in legumes. Therefore, quinoa is the perfect complement for both grains and legumes—or perfect all on its own.

Quinoa has more riboflavin, alpha tocopherol, and carotenes than wheat, rice, or barley. One cup of cooked quinoa is a good source of the minerals magnesium, zinc, copper, and iron. It also provides the B vitamins pyridoxine, pantothenic acid, folate, biotin, thiamin, and niacin.

Health and Quinoa

Vegetarians

Quinoa is an excellent source of protein for the individual who eats no animal products or who has to limit the amount of animal protein they consume. Unlike other grains, it is a complete protein, containing high amounts of all the essential amino acids.

The Incas encouraged their pregnant and lactating women to eat quinoa every day. This is a smart idea for the woman who limits the amount of animal protein she eats. Quinoa is also an excellent grain choice for vegetarian teenagers and children, who have high protein needs due to fast growth.

High Cholesterol

Quinoa contains bitter-tasting compounds called saponins. Although much of the saponin coating on the seed is washed away before packaging, some still remains. Research studies indicate that diets rich in saponins reduce the plasma cholesterol by 16 to 24%. Quinoa also contains phytic acid, a compound that may also reduce cholesterol levels.

Cancer Prevention

Phytic acid and saponins, the same two phytochemicals that reduce cholesterol levels, also appear to prevent some forms of cancer. Quinoa as a whole grain is also a good source of fiber, and high-fiber diets are associated with reduced risks of colon and rectal cancer.

How to Use Quinoa

Quinoa has a mild flavor and can be substituted in recipes for couscous, bulgur, buckwheat, or millet. It can be used in stuffings, soups, and puddings, as a topping for salads, or as hot breakfast porridge.

Quinoa is rich in oil, so it has a limited shelf life. In warm weather, store quinoa in a sealed container in the refrigerator to prevent the grain from becoming rancid.

Recipes

Basic Cooking Instructions

Place quinoa in a strainer and rinse thoroughly under running water or place in a pot and wash by running water over the pot. This removes the bitter saponins that coat each grain. To each 1 cup of quinoa, add 2 cups of water and steam for 15 minutes. When quinoa is done the grain will be translucent. The ring of germ will be visible as a "tail."

Quinoa can be toasted before cooking to give it a nutty flavor. Place the grain in a hot, dry skillet and toast the grain until it is golden brown. Some of the grain will "pop" during toasting, so be prepared for these hot flying missiles. Be careful not to overtoast the grain.

2 cups water, juice, or broth
1 cup quinoa
Salt to taste

Plastic Steamers

Fill reservoir to maximum with water and turn on machine. Add quinoa and cooking liquid to rice bowl and steam for 30 minutes. Season and serve.

Metal Steamers

Coat rice bowl with nonstick spray. Add quinoa and cooking liquid plus an additional 1 cup of water. Let steam for 5 minutes after machine switches to warm. Season and serve.

Serves 4

Nutrition Facts	
Serving Size 1.499 ounces (42.50g)	
Servings Per Container 4	
Amount Per Serving	
Calories 159 Calories from Fat 22	
	% *Daily Value**
Total Fat 2g	3%
Saturated Fat 0g	0%
Cholesterol 0mg	0%
Sodium 9mg	0%
Total Carbohydrate 29g	10%
Dietary Fiber 2g	8%
Sugars 0g	
Protein 6g	
Vitamin A 0%	Vitamin C 0%
Calcium 2%	Iron 21%

*Percent Daily Values are based on a 2,000 calorie diet. Your daily values may be higher or lower depending on your calorie needs.

Breakfast Quinoa

Kids love these darling little grains with a tail. Offer several toppings such as shredded coconut, raisins, and nuts and let kids make their own creations with this dish. They love to eat something they've made themselves.

1 cup quinoa
2 cups water
2 tablespoons maple syrup
¼ cup shredded coconut, toasted
Pineapple bits (garnish)
Salt to taste

Plastic Steamers
Fill reservoir to maximum with water and turn on machine. Add grain, water, and syrup to rice bowl and let steam for 30 minutes. Season to taste and sprinkle each serving with 1 tablespoon coconut and pineapple bits.

Metal Steamers
Coat rice bowl with nonstick spray. Add all ingredients to steamer bowl and an additional ½ cup water. Cook until machine turns off. Let steam on warm for 5 more minutes. Season to taste and sprinkle each serving with 1 tablespoon coconut and pineapple bits.

Serves 4

Nutrition Facts	
Serving Size 2.014 ounces (57.09g)	
Servings Per Container 4	
Amount Per Serving	
Calories 201 Calories from Fat 37	
	% *Daily Value**
Total Fat 4g	6%
Saturated Fat 2g	10%
Cholesterol 0mg	0%
Sodium 11mg	1%
Total Carbohydrate 36g	12%
Dietary Fiber 3g	12%
Sugars 0g	
Protein 6g	
Vitamin A 0%	Vitamin C 0%
Calcium 3%	Iron 23%

*Percent Daily Values are based on a 2,000 calorie diet. Your daily values may be higher or lower depending on your calorie needs.

Quinoa and Millet Pilaf

Be creative with vegetable choices in any of the pilaf recipes. Use whatever you have in the fridge, or choose bright-colored vegetables such as red bell peppers or purple onion.

2 cups water
½ cup quinoa
½ cup millet
1 teaspoon olive oil
½ medium onion, chopped
½ cup carrot, chopped
½ teaspoon ground cumin
Salt to taste

Plastic Steamers
Fill water reservoir to maximum with water and turn on machine. Add all ingredients to steamer bowl and cook for 45 minutes. Season and serve.

Metal Steamers
Coat rice bowl with nonstick spray. Add all ingredients to steamer bowl with an additional 1 cup of water. After machine turns off, let grain steam for 5 minutes on warm. Season and serve.

Serves 4

Nutrition Facts	
Serving Size 2.387 ounces (67.66g)	
Servings Per Container 4	

Amount Per Serving	
Calories 192 Calories from Fat 31	

	% *Daily Value**
Total Fat 3g	5%
Saturated Fat 0g	0%
Cholesterol 0mg	0%
Sodium 6mg	0%
Total Carbohydrate 35g	12%
Dietary Fiber 5g	20%
Sugars 1g	
Protein 6g	

Vitamin A 0%	Vitamin C 2%
Calcium 1%	Iron 15%

*Percent Daily Values are based on a 2,000 calorie diet. Your daily values may be higher or lower depending on your calorie needs.

Quinoa Pudding

Your choice of sweetener will be the overriding flavor of this pudding. Molasses gives a caramel color and rich flavor, honey a light sweetness, and date sugar a traditional dessert flavor.

2 cups cooked quinoa
3 cups lowfat milk or soy milk
3 eggs, slightly beaten
½ cup raisins
⅓ cup molasses
½ cup chopped almonds
½ teaspoon cinnamon
1 teaspoon vanilla
Salt to taste

Combine ingredients and pour into baking dish or individual custard cups. Bake in 350° oven for 45 minutes or until set. Serve warm.

Serves 8

Nutrition Facts	
Serving Size 5.749 ounces (163.0g)	
Servings Per Container 8	

Amount Per Serving

Calories 252   Calories from Fat 75

	% Daily Value*
Total Fat 8g	12%
Saturated Fat 2g	10%
Cholesterol 84mg	28%
Sodium 89mg	4%
Total Carbohydrate 36g	12%
Dietary Fiber 2g	8%
Sugars 11g	
Protein 10g	

Vitamin A 9%	Vitamin C 2%
Calcium 25%	Iron 27%

*Percent Daily Values are based on a 2,000 calorie diet. Your daily values may be higher or lower depending on your calorie needs.

Quinoa Tabbouleh Salad

Fresh parsley, mint, and lemon juice are the bright flavors that make this Lebanese dish so popular. The quinoa mingles beautifully with these flavors.

1 cup cooked quinoa
1 green onion, minced
1¼ cups minced parsley
½ cup minced fresh mint
1 tablespoon lemon juice
1 tablespoon olive oil
1 teaspoon cumin
White pepper to taste

Combine all ingredients and chill.

Serves 4

Nutrition Facts

Serving Size 2.656 ounces (75.29g)
Servings Per Container 4

Amount Per Serving

Calories 129   Calories from Fat 45

	% Daily Value*
Total Fat 5g	8%
Saturated Fat 1g	5%
Cholesterol 0mg	0%
Sodium 16mg	1%
Total Carbohydrate 18g	6%
Dietary Fiber 2g	8%
Sugars 0g	
Protein 4g	

Vitamin A 23%	Vitamin C 80%
Calcium 9%	Iron 24%

*Percent Daily Values are based on a 2,000 calorie diet. Your daily values may be higher or lower depending on your calorie needs.

Scorched Onion Quinoa

Onions become caramelized and the natural sweet flavors are released when they are sautéed. This makes a good topping for salads.

⅔ cup water
½ cup onions, chopped
⅓ cup quinoa
1 tablespoon olive oil

Add olive oil to skillet and heat oil. Add quinoa and onion and sauté 4 to 5 minutes until grain is a light brown but onions are not burned. Steam as described below. Cool and sprinkle on top of salads.

Plastic Steamers
Fill reservoir to maximum with water and turn on machine. Add sautéed mixture to steamer bowl and steam for 40 minutes.

Metal Steamers
Coat rice bowl with nonstick spray. Add sautéed mixture to steamer bowl with 1 cup of additional water and turn machine on.

Serves 4

Nutrition Facts	
Serving Size 1.319 ounces (37.40g)	
Servings Per Container 4	
Amount Per Serving	
Calories 90 Calories from Fat 38	
	% *Daily Value**
Total Fat 4g	6%
Saturated Fat 1g	5%
Cholesterol 0mg	0%
Sodium 4mg	0%
Total Carbohydrate 11g	4%
Dietary Fiber 1g	4%
Sugars 1g	
Protein 2g	
Vitamin A 0%	Vitamin C 2%
Calcium 1%	Iron 7%

*Percent Daily Values are based on a 2,000 calorie diet. Your daily values may be higher or lower depending on your calorie needs.

Quick Southwest Quinoa

This is one of our favorite recipes because it's so easy, and fresh cilantro gives this dish a real Western flavor.

2 cups cooked quinoa
1 cup fresh salsa
¼ cup chopped cilantro
Lemon and fresh chopped tomato (optional)

Mix cooked quinoa in a bowl with salsa and cilantro. Serve warm or cold. Squeeze ½ of a lemon on top for a fresh, tangy addition.

Serves 4

Nutrition Facts	
Serving Size 3.827 ounces (108.5g)	
Servings Per Container 4	
Amount Per Serving	
Calories 170 Calories from Fat 22	
	% Daily Value*
Total Fat 2g	3%
Saturated Fat 2g	10%
Cholesterol 2mg	1%
Sodium 458mg	19%
Total Carbohydrate 32g	11%
Dietary Fiber 3g	12%
Sugars 0g	
Protein 6g	
Vitamin A 9%	Vitamin C 39%
Calcium 3%	Iron 24%

*Percent Daily Values are based on a 2,000 calorie diet. Your daily values may be higher or lower depending on your calorie needs.

Cashew Quinoa

Nuts and raisins give you something to really sink your teeth into here.

2 cups water
1 cup quinoa
¼ cup cashews
¼ cup raisins
⅛ teaspoon cinnamon
Salt to taste

Plastic Steamers
Fill reservoir to maximum with water and turn on machine. Add all ingredients and steam for 40 to 45 minutes.

Metal Steamers
Coat rice bowl with nonstick spray. Add all ingredients plus an additional 1 cup of water. After machine turns off, let grain steam on warm for 5 minutes.

Serves 4

Nutrition Facts	
Serving Size 2.124 ounces (60.21g)	
Servings Per Container 4	
Amount Per Serving	
Calories 236 Calories from Fat 58	
	% *Daily Value**
Total Fat 6g	9%
Saturated Fat 1g	5%
Cholesterol 0mg	0%
Sodium 11mg	1%
Total Carbohydrate 39g	13%
Dietary Fiber 3g	12%
Sugars 6g	
Protein 7g	
Vitamin A 0%	Vitamin C 0%
Calcium 3%	Iron 25%

*Percent Daily Values are based on a 2,000 calorie diet. Your daily values may be higher or lower depending on your calorie needs.

Quinoa with Bulgur

Other quinoa or bulgur recipes can be altered using this combination of 50/50 quinoa/bulgur. Be creative and have fun!

2 cups water
½ cup quinoa
½ cup bulgur
1 teaspoon soy sauce

Plastic Steamers
Fill reservoir to maximum with water and turn on machine. Add all ingredients to steamer bowl and steam for 40 minutes.

Metal Steamers
Coat rice bowl with nonstick spray. Add all ingredients plus 1 additional cup of water. After machine turns off, let grain steam on warm for 5 minutes before serving.

Serves 4

Nutrition Facts	
Serving Size 1.409 ounces (39.93g)	
Servings Per Container 4	
Amount Per Serving	
Calories 139 Calories from Fat 13	
	% *Daily Value**
Total Fat 1g	2%
Saturated Fat 0g	0%
Cholesterol 0mg	0%
Sodium 59mg	2%
Total Carbohydrate 28g	9%
Dietary Fiber 5g	20%
Sugars 0g	
Protein 5g	
Vitamin A 0%	Vitamin C 0%
Calcium 1%	Iron 13%

*Percent Daily Values are based on a 2,000 calorie diet. Your daily values may be higher or lower depending on your calorie needs.

CHAPTER 13

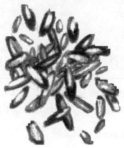

Rice (Oryza sativa var.)

The range of specialty and brown rices offers a variety of shapes, sizes, colors, and defining sweet flavors.

Rice is one of the oldest food crops and probably originated in Southeast Asia. Archeologists have found evidence in Thailand that rice was cultivated for food by about 5000 B.C. In China there was a ceremony dating back to 3000 B.C. in which the emperor and princess honored the rice planting by sowing a handful of seed. Rice reached the American Colonies during the 1600s.

Rice is still one of the world's most important food crops. It is the staple food for over half the world's population and provides over half the daily calories for many people in Asia.

What Is Rice?

Rice is a true cereal grain that is tan in color and has a nutlike flavor. When cooked, the outer portion is slightly crunchy while the inner portion is tender.

Unlike other grains, rice grows best in shallow water and thrives in warm, wet climates. Farmers usually flood rice fields to supply the growing plants with moisture and to kill weeds and other pests.

Nutrition and Rice

Over a hundred years ago Dr. K. Takaki, a Japanese physician, suspected that something in the refined rice diet of his country was causing people to develop beriberi. Beriberi is a disease characterized by degeneration of the nervous system and heart failure. In an experiment, Japanese sailors were fed either the usual polished rice diet or a British diet of whole grain barley, milk, meat, and vegetables. The group consuming the British diet did not develop the beriberi that the group eating the traditional Japanese diet did.

As the use of refined cereals became more widespread, beriberi became a major health problem. Eventually it was recognized that some agent in rice bran miraculously cured beriberi. In the middle of the 1920s, one teaspoon of the agent was extracted from a ton of bran, but it was 1936 before this agent was chemically defined and named thiamin or vitamin B-1. Today, thiamin is added back to refined grains and beriberi is rarely seen. You, however, can get your thiamin naturally from brown rice.

Rice contains more lysine, the limiting amino acid in true cereals, and so it is a good source of protein. Brown rice is also a good source of other B vitamins such as niacin and pyridoxine. Rice bran and rice polish are concentrated sources of these vitamins.

Magnesium and iron are found in brown rice, but the phytic acid present in the bran may decrease their bioavailability. To increase the absorption of minerals from brown rice, always include a source of vitamin C with the meal. A list of foods rich in vitamin C can be found in chapter 5.

Brown rice is also an excellent source of insoluble fiber.

Health and Rice

Rice is an excellent substitute for all grains and can be found in many different forms. Eating rice is a wonderful way for individuals who are allergic or sensitive to wheat or gluten to reap the benefits of whole grains.

Baby Food (cereal)

Rice is the most frequently recommended cereal for babies under the age of one year because it rarely causes allergies. Directions for making baby cereal can be found in chapter 5.

Celiac Disease (Gluten Intolerance)

Celiac disease is an inherited inability to tolerate two of the amino acids found in the gluten of barley, oats, buckwheat, wheat, rye, and triticale. When grains that contain these amino acids are eaten, an immune reaction destroys the lining of the small intestine, making absorption impossible. If sufferers do not follow a prolamin- and gliadin-free diet, they starve to death. Researchers believe that celiac disease can also cause cancer of the gastrointestinal tract. Rice can substitute for almost any grain in the recipes in this book. A list of ingredients that gluten-sensitive individuals must avoid is found at the end of this chapter.

Constipation

Wheat bran is the grain usually recommended to increase the fiber content of the diet and prevent constipation. If you are allergic to wheat or suffer from gluten intolerance, rice bran can substitute for wheat bran. When rice bran was given to volunteers, it caused an increase in intestinal transit time that was greater than with a larger amount of wheat bran. Add a tablespoon of rice bran to your morning cereal to prevent constipation and the hemorrhoids it can promote.

Heartburn

Studies show that rice reduces acidity in the stomach and aids in reducing discomfort due to esophageal reflux, the splashing of stomach acid into the esophagus.

High Cholesterol

Although brown rice is low in soluble fiber, it has demonstrated an ability to decrease serum-cholesterol levels. Some of the substances found in brown rice that are suspected of contributing to this effect include tocotrienols, a form of vitamin E; oryzanols; beta sitosterol; and rice wax. Since these substances are concentrated in the oil of the bran, milled or white rice is not effective.

Irritable Bowel Syndrome (IBS)

IBS is a disease in which the patient suffers from alternating bouts of constipation and diarrhea. Food sensitivities appear to worsen symptoms in some individuals. Rice is the grain least likely to upset the irritable colon. Grains such as wheat, oats, and to a lesser extent barley should be avoided for a trial period, to determine whether they are worsening symptoms.

Kidney Stones

Dr. Ebisuno and coworkers treated 182 calcium stone formers with rice bran therapy. The subjects were given 10 grams of rice bran twice daily after meals. This drastically reduced new stone formation, with 61% remaining in remission during therapy. If you suffer from recurrent kidney stones, ask your physician about trying this treatment and then get out your grain steamer.

How to Buy Rice

About twenty-five species of *Oryza* furnish all the rice of the world. Thousands of strains or varieties of rice are known today.

Rice can be purchased in the form of whole kernels, ground kernels, flour, or bran. It is often cheaper to buy rice in bulk. Do not buy rice from bulk containers, however, if you are allergic or sensitive to other cereal grains. The rice can become contaminated with other grain through shared scoops.

Brown Rice

Brown rice is the rice kernel with just the hull removed. The nutrient-rich bran and germ layer are left intact. This is the most nutritious form of rice.

Polished or White Rice

Polishing is an abrasive process that removes the bran and most of the germ. White rice is missing the bran, germ, vitamins, and minerals found in brown rice.

Converted Rice

Converted rice is white rice that has been steeped in water, steamed, and then dried again before milling. This causes many of the B vitamins present in the bran and germ to diffuse into the endosperm. However, converted rice is still a refined product that is missing all of the benefits found in the bran, and we do not recommend the use of it.

Quick Cooking or Instant Brown Rice

Instant brown rice is made by partially cooking and then fissuring the grain. It can then be freeze dried, puffed, rolled, or microwaved. Instant rice cooks faster than regular brown rice, but it lacks flavor and texture.

Brown Rice Farina

Brown rice farina is made by stone grinding brown rice. Farina makes a creamy hot cereal. Most of the rice farina available in supermarkets is made from polished white rice. Make sure that you buy *brown* rice farina, which is available at health food stores and through the mail order companies listed in the back of the book.

Strains of Rice

Basmati

Basmati is a strain that is grown in India and Pakistan and prized for its wonderful aroma and flavor. It is aged for a year after harvesting to develop its flavor.

Texamati

Texamati is similar to Basmati in aroma and flavor. It is grown in Texas.

Wehani

Wehani is a fragrant rice grown in California that smells like hot, buttered peanuts. It has a reddish color and a nutty flavor.

Black and Red Rice

There are a number of rare, exotic strains of black and red rice grown in California. Lundberg Farms has trademarked two varieties: Black Japonica and Mahogany. Lundberg Farms also makes a "limited edition" Christmas blend that is a treat we look forward to. (Information about ordering these rices can be found in the suppliers listing at the end of this book.)

Long-Grain Brown Rice

Long-grain rice is a perfect all-purpose rice. It cooks up fluffy and separate.

Medium-Grain Brown Rice

Medium-grain rice is shorter and wider than long grain. It is bland in taste and cooks up soft. Medium grain can be substituted for long grain in any recipe.

Short-Grain Brown Rice

Short-grain rice is shorter and wider than medium. It has a higher percentage of starch, so it cooks up soft and tends to stick together. Short-grain rice is perfect for rice puddings and desserts.

How to Use Rice

Rice can be used to make steamed puddings, pilafs, casseroles, hot breakfast cereals, or just on its own. There are enough different varieties of rice and ways of preparing it that you could eat rice every day of the year—as much of the world actually does—and never tire of it.

Because brown rice includes the oil-containing bran, it can go rancid if stored improperly. Store your brown rice in a cool, dry place in a sealed container for up to one year.

Recipes

Basic Cooking Instructions

Rinse rice in water and remove any debris before adding to rice cooker. All grain steamers come with instructions on how to cook rice in that particular machine. We found that most instructions underestimated the amount of time and water it took to make brown rice. Make three or four days' worth of unseasoned rice at once and reheat as necessary.

1 cup brown rice
1 cup water, juice, or broth
Salt to taste

Plastic Steamers
Fill reservoir with maximum amount of water and turn on machine. Add rice and water to rice bowl and steam for 50 to 60 minutes. Season and serve.

Metal Steamers
Coat rice bowl with nonstick spray. Add rice, water, and an additional 1½ cups water. Turn machine on. After machine switches to warm, add salt and let steam for 10 minutes.

Serves 4

Nutrition Facts	
Serving Size 3.439 ounces (97.50g)	
Servings Per Container 4	
Amount Per Serving	
Calories 108 Calories from Fat 8	
	% Daily Value*
Total Fat 1g	2%
Saturated Fat 0g	0%
Cholesterol 0mg	0%
Sodium 4mg	0%
Total Carbohydrate 22g	7%
Dietary Fiber 2g	8%
Sugars 0g	
Protein 3g	
Vitamin A 0%	Vitamin C 0%
Calcium 1%	Iron 2%

*Percent Daily Values are based on a 2,000 calorie diet. Your daily values may be higher or lower depending on your calorie needs.

Breakfast Rice

A warm, comforting way to start your day. The wonderful aroma of the hot berries is a real eye-opener.

1 cup brown rice farina
½ cup vanilla soy milk or lowfat cow's milk
½ cup water
1 cup frozen unsweetened strawberries
Salt to taste
Brown rice syrup

Plastic Steamers
Fill reservoir with minimum amount of water and turn on machine. Add rice, milk, water, and strawberries to rice bowl and steam for 20 minutes. Add salt to taste and drizzle with rice syrup.

Metal Steamers
Coat rice bowl with nonstick spray. Add rice, milk, water, and strawberries to rice bowl with an additional ½ cup of water. Cook until machine turns off and let steam for a few more minutes on warm. Add salt to taste and drizzle with rice syrup.

Serves 4

Nutrition Facts	
Serving Size 4.065 ounces (115.3g)	
Servings Per Container 4	

Amount Per Serving	
Calories 204 Calories from Fat 17	

	% *Daily Value**
Total Fat 2g	3%
Saturated Fat 0g	0%
Cholesterol 0mg	0%
Sodium 18mg	1%
Total Carbohydrate 42g	14%
Dietary Fiber 2g	8%
Sugars 2g	
Protein 4g	

Vitamin A 6%	Vitamin C 25%
Calcium 5%	Iron 7%

*Percent Daily Values are based on a 2,000 calorie diet. Your daily values may be higher or lower depending on your calorie needs.

Nutty Rice Pilaf

Experiment with different types of rice for variations on this recipe.

2 cups onions, chopped
1 cup water
1 cup brown long grain rice
¼ cup slivered almonds or pine nuts
2 sprigs fresh chopped thyme or ½ teaspoon dried
1 bay leaf

Plastic Steamers
Fill reservoir with maximum amount of water and turn on machine. Add all ingredients to rice bowl and steam for 50 to 60 minutes. Season and serve.

Metal Steamers
Coat rice bowl with nonstick spray. Add all ingredients and an additional 1½ cups water. Turn machine on. After machine switches to warm, add salt and let steam for 10 minutes.

Serves 4

Nutrition Facts	
Serving Size 4.713 ounces (133.6g)	
Servings Per Container 4	

Amount Per Serving	
Calories 244 Calories from Fat 47	

	% *Daily Value**
Total Fat 5g	8%
Saturated Fat 1g	5%
Cholesterol 0mg	0%
Sodium 7mg	0%
Total Carbohydrate 44g	15%
Dietary Fiber 5g	20%
Sugars 3g	
Protein 6g	

Vitamin A 0%	Vitamin C 8%
Calcium 4%	Iron 7%

*Percent Daily Values are based on a 2,000 calorie diet. Your daily values may be higher or lower depending on your calorie needs.

Magic Rice

This is a great way to sneak the dreaded veggie into your vege-phobic offspring. Just make them disappear (the vegetables, not the kids). Fresh carrot juice or tomato juice works best.

1 cup long-grain brown rice
1½ cups fresh vegetable juice
½ cup sultana raisins
Salt to taste

Plastic Steamers
Fill reservoir to maximum with water and turn on machine. Add rice and juice to rice bowl. Steam for 50 to 60 minutes. Ten minutes before rice is done, add raisins and salt.

Metal Steamers
Coat rice bowl with nonstick spray. Add rice and juice and an additional 1 cup of water. After machine turns off, add raisins and salt and steam for 10 minutes.

Serves 4

Nutrition Facts	
Serving Size 4.524 ounces (128.3g)	
Servings Per Container 4	
Amount Per Serving	
Calories 248 Calories from Fat 13	
	% *Daily Value**
Total Fat 1g	2%
Saturated Fat 0g	0%
Cholesterol 0mg	0%
Sodium 20mg	1%
Total Carbohydrate 55g	18%
Dietary Fiber 4g	16%
Sugars 2g	
Protein 4g	
Vitamin A 10%	Vitamin C 23%
Calcium 3%	Iron 8%

*Percent Daily Values are based on a 2,000 calorie diet. Your daily values may be higher or lower depending on your calorie needs.

Rice Bran Cereal

There is no better way to start your day when you are trying to lower your cholesterol levels. The rice bran and soy milk help to decrease cholesterol levels. This cereal is also effective in promoting regularity.

1 cup water
¾ cup rice farina
½ cup pitted prunes, chopped
¼ cup rice bran
2 tablespoons date sugar
1 tablespoon ground flaxseeds
Salt to taste
Soy milk or lowfat cow's milk

Plastic Steamers
Fill reservoir with water and turn on machine. Add ingredients to rice bowl and steam for 15 to 20 minutes. Season to taste and serve with milk.

Metal Steamers
Coat rice bowl with nonstick spray. Add all ingredients plus an additional ½ cup of water and cook until machine turns off. Let steam for a few minutes on warm before serving. Season to taste and serve with milk.

Serves 4

Nutrition Facts	
Serving Size 2.387 ounces (67.67g)	
Servings Per Container 4	
Amount Per Serving	
Calories 220 Calories from Fat 30	
	% *Daily Value**
Total Fat 3g	5%
Saturated Fat 1g	5%
Cholesterol 0mg	0%
Sodium 5mg	0%
Total Carbohydrate 46g	15%
Dietary Fiber 4g	16%
Sugars 4g	
Protein 5g	
Vitamin A 3%	Vitamin C 1%
Calcium 3%	Iron 13%

*Percent Daily Values are based on a 2,000 calorie diet. Your daily values may be higher or lower depending on your calorie needs.

Indian Rice

East Indian recipes have been made for five thousand years.
That's a lot of years of perfecting.

1 teaspoon sunflower oil
½ teaspoon mustard seeds
½ teaspoon cumin seeds
1 cup water
1 cup basmati rice
¼ teaspoon freshly ground black pepper
Salt to taste

In a small frying pan, heat oil and add mustard seeds and
cumin seeds. When the mustard seeds pop, they are ready to
be added to the rest of the ingredients in the machine's cooking pan.

Plastic Steamers
Fill reservoir to maximum with
water and turn on machine.
Add all ingredients to rice bowl.
Steam for 50 to 60 minutes.
Season and serve.

Metal Steamers
Coat rice bowl with nonstick
spray. Add all ingredients plus
an additional 1½ cups of water.
After machine turns off, steam
on warm for 5 minutes. Season
and serve.

Serves 4

Nutrition Facts	
Serving Size 1.700 ounces (48.19g)	
Servings Per Container 4	
Amount Per Serving	
Calories 184 Calories from Fat 24	
	% *Daily Value**
Total Fat 3g	5%
Saturated Fat 0g	0%
Cholesterol 0mg	0%
Sodium 4mg	0%
Total Carbohydrate 36g	12%
Dietary Fiber 3g	12%
Sugars 0g	
Protein 4g	
Vitamin A 0%	Vitamin C 0%
Calcium 1%	Iron 5%

*Percent Daily Values are based on a
2,000 calorie diet. Your daily values
may be higher or lower depending on
your calorie needs.

Basmati Rice

Adding whole spices, which are removed after cooking, lends a mild flavor to the dish and is often more acceptable to children than flecks of mysterious spices.

1 cup water
1 cup brown basmati rice
3 whole cloves
5 green or black peppercorns
1 cinnamon stick
½ cup fresh or frozen baby peas
1 tablespoon sliced almonds, toasted
½ teaspoon fresh lemon juice

Plastic Steamers
Fill water reservoir to maximum and turn on machine. Steam for 1 hour. When done, remove cloves, peppercorns, and cinnamon stick.

Metal Steamers
Coat rice bowl with nonstick spray. Add all ingredients plus 1½ cups of water and start machine. When done, remove cloves, peppercorns, and cinnamon stick.

Serves 4

Nutrition Facts	
Serving Size 2.503 ounces (70.95g)	
Servings Per Container 4	
Amount Per Serving	
Calories 208 Calories from Fat 28	
	% *Daily Value**
Total Fat 3g	5%
Saturated Fat 0g	0%
Cholesterol 0mg	0%
Sodium 22mg	1%
Total Carbohydrate 40g	13%
Dietary Fiber 4g	16%
Sugars 1g	
Protein 6g	
Vitamin A 1%	Vitamin C 4%
Calcium 3%	Iron 6%

*Percent Daily Values are based on a 2,000 calorie diet. Your daily values may be higher or lower depending on your calorie needs.

Dessert Pie Crust

This a great use for leftover rice. Perfect shell for quiches, casseroles, or desserts.

2 cups well-cooked short-grain brown rice
2 eggs, lightly beaten
2 tablespoons date sugar or Succanet
1 teaspoon nutmeg, pumpkin pie spice, or herb of your choice
Salt to taste

Mix ingredients together. Coat pie pan with nonstick spray and press rice mixture into plate. Bake at 350° for 10 minutes or until golden brown. Fill with your favorite dessert filling.

Makes two pie crusts

Nutrition Facts	
Serving Size 5.202 ounces (147.5g)	
Servings Per Container 2	
Amount Per Serving	
Calories 424 Calories from Fat 72	
	% *Daily Value**
Total Fat 8g	12%
Saturated Fat 2g	10%
Cholesterol 213mg	71%
Sodium 600mg	25%
Total Carbohydrate 74g	25%
Dietary Fiber 2g	8%
Sugars 0g	
Protein 13g	
Vitamin A 9%	Vitamin C 0%
Calcium 6%	Iron 13%

*Percent Daily Values are based on a 2,000 calorie diet. Your daily values may be higher or lower depending on your calorie needs.

Javanese Spiced Rice

This bright, beautiful dish will romance you with the flavors of the East. The quantity of hot spices will have a therapeutic effect, as they all increase circulation.

1 cup long-grain brown rice
1 cup lowfat chicken broth
⅛ cup chopped green onions
1 tablespoon peanut oil
¼ teaspoon sesame oil
¼ large red onion, diced
⅛ green pepper, diced
⅛ yellow pepper, diced
½ small jalapeno chili, seeded, minced
¾ teaspoon turmeric
¼ teaspoon cayenne
⅛ teaspoon cinnamon
Salt to taste

Plastic Steamers
Fill water reservoir to maximum and turn on machine. Add all ingredients to steamer bowl and cook for 50 to 60 minutes. Serve with a dollop of chilled lowfat yogurt.

Metal Steamers
Coat rice bowl with nonstick spray. Add all ingredients plus 1½ cups of water and start machine. Serve with a dollop of chilled lowfat yogurt.

Serves 4

Nutrition Facts		
Serving Size 4.521 ounces (128.2g)		
Servings Per Container 4		
Amount Per Serving		
Calories 225 Calories from Fat 51		
		% *Daily Value**
Total Fat 6g		9%
Saturated Fat 1g		5%
Cholesterol 0mg		0%
Sodium 158mg		7%
Total Carbohydrate 39g		13%
Dietary Fiber 3g		12%
Sugars 0g		
Protein 5g		
Vitamin A 1%		Vitamin C 31%
Calcium 1%		Iron 6%

*Percent Daily Values are based on a 2,000 calorie diet. Your daily values may be higher or lower depending on your calorie needs.

Green Rice with Sunflower Seeds

These greens are full of chlorophyll and fresh flavor. Serve this warm or cooled in the summer.

1 cup lowfat chicken broth
1½ cups fresh spinach, chopped
1 cup long-grain brown rice
¾ cup chopped green onions
½ cup parsley, finely chopped
¼ cup celery leaves, chopped
2 tablespoons sunflower seeds
½ teaspoon pepper
Salt to taste

Plastic Steamers
Fill water reservoir to maximum and turn on machine. Add all ingredients to steamer bowl and cook for 50 to 60 minutes.

Metal Steamers
Coat rice bowl with nonstick spray. Add all ingredients plus 1½ cups additional water and start machine.

Serves 4

Nutrition Facts	
Serving Size 6.616 ounces (187.6g)	
Servings Per Container 4	
Amount Per Serving	
Calories 216 Calories from Fat 38	
	% *Daily Value**
Total Fat 4g	6%
Saturated Fat 1g	5%
Cholesterol 0mg	0%
Sodium 180mg	8%
Total Carbohydrate 39g	13%
Dietary Fiber 4g	16%
Sugars 0g	
Protein 8g	
Vitamin A 18%	Vitamin C 23%
Calcium 4%	Iron 13%

*Percent Daily Values are based on a 2,000 calorie diet. Your daily values may be higher or lower depending on your calorie needs.

Italian Rice

This dish is a nice accompaniment to broiled chicken breast, French bread, and wine.

1 cup vegetable or lowfat chicken broth
1 cup brown rice
3 ounces sun-dried tomatoes
¼ cup red wine
4 green onions, finely chopped
4 cloves, minced
1 teaspoon dried basil
Salt to taste

Plastic Steamers
Fill water reservoir to maximum and turn on machine. Mix all ingredients in steamer bowl and cook until all broth is absorbed, about 50 to 60 minutes. Serve warm.

Metal Steamers
Coat rice bowl with nonstick spray. Mix all ingredients in rice bowl, plus 1½ cups additional water, and cook until all broth is absorbed. Serve warm.

Serves 4

Nutrition Facts
Serving Size 7.542 ounces (213.8g)
Servings Per Container 4

Amount Per Serving	
Calories 266 Calories from Fat 20	

	% *Daily Value**
Total Fat 2g	3%
Saturated Fat 1g	5%
Cholesterol 0mg	0%
Sodium 430mg	18%
Total Carbohydrate 52g	17%
Dietary Fiber 4g	16%
Sugars 0g	
Protein 9g	

Vitamin A 112%	Vitamin C 42%
Calcium 6%	Iron 12%

*Percent Daily Values are based on a 2,000 calorie diet. Your daily values may be higher or lower depending on your calorie needs.

Singapore Rice Salad

This salad makes a great summer party dish. Make it the day before and warm it in the microwave.

2 cups water
2 cups long grain brown rice
1 red bell pepper, diced
½ cup sliced green onions
½ cup carrots, shredded
¼ cup teriyaki sauce
1 tablespoon lime juice
½ cup pineapple tidbits, drained
1 cup diced cucumber

Garnish: chopped cilantro, peanuts or cashews, cucumber slices

Plastic Steamers

Fill water reservoir to maximum and turn on machine. Add all ingredients except cucumber and pineapple pieces to steamer bowl. Cook for 50 minutes and add cucumber and pineapple. Garnish and serve warm.

Metal Steamers

Coat rice bowl with nonstick spray. Add all ingredients plus 1½ cups additional water. Cook until all liquid is absorbed. Add cucumber and pineapple and warm for an additional 10 minutes. Garnish and serve warm.

Serves 8

Nutrition Facts	
Serving Size 4.021 ounces (114.0g)	
Servings Per Container 8	
Amount Per Serving	
Calories 192 Calories from Fat 13	
	% *Daily Value**
Total Fat 1g	2%
Saturated Fat 0g	0%
Cholesterol 0mg	0%
Sodium 351mg	15%
Total Carbohydrate 40g	13%
Dietary Fiber 4g	16%
Sugars 2g	
Protein 5g	
Vitamin A 20%	Vitamin C 32%
Calcium 2%	Iron 5%

*Percent Daily Values are based on a 2,000 calorie diet. Your daily values may be higher or lower depending on your calorie needs.

Puerto Rican Rice and Beans (Arroz con Habichuelas)

This healthy combination of proteins really sticks to your ribs.

1 cup vegetable or lowfat chicken broth
1 cup long-grain brown rice
½ cup chopped onion
2 cloves garlic, peeled and chopped
1 large red bell pepper, cored, seeded, and diced
1 jalapeno pepper, seeded and diced
1 teaspoon olive oil
1 8-ounce can pinto beans, drained
1 15-ounce can peeled plum tomatoes, drained and juice
   reserved
2 teaspoons dried oregano
½ teaspoon black pepper
2 tablespoons capers
Salt to taste
3 tablespoons fresh, chopped cilantro

Plastic Steamers
Fill water reservoir to maximum and turn on machine. Mix broth and rice in steamer bowl and start the cooking process. Then sauté onion, garlic, bell pepper, and jalapeno pepper in oil in a frying pan for 5 minutes. When onions become translucent, add to steamer with pinto beans, tomatoes, oregano, black pepper, and capers. Steam for 50 to 60 minutes. Season, garnish with fresh cilantro, and serve warm.

Metal Steamers
Coat rice bowl with nonstick spray. Mix the broth and rice and 1½ cups additional water in the rice bowl and start the cooking process. Then sauté onion, garlic, bell pepper, and jalapeno pepper in oil in a frying pan for 5 minutes. When onions become translucent, add to steamer with pinto beans,

tomatoes, oregano, black pepper, and capers. Cook until all liquid is absorbed. Season, garnish with fresh cilantro, and serve warm.

Serves 4

```
Nutrition Facts
Serving Size 13.23 ounces (375.0g)
Servings Per Container 4

Amount Per Serving
Calories 275   Calories from Fat 32

                        % Daily Value*
Total Fat 4g                     6%
   Saturated Fat 1g              5%
Cholesterol 0mg                  0%
Sodium 649mg                    27%
Total Carbohydrate 53g          18%
   Dietary Fiber 5g             20%
   Sugars 1g
Protein 10g

Vitamin A 8%          Vitamin C 78%
Calcium 7%                 Iron 17%

*Percent Daily Values are based on a
2,000 calorie diet. Your daily values
may be higher or lower depending on
your calorie needs.
```

Saffron Rice

Saffron threads are expensive, but they keep for years. They have a most unusual flavor that really grows on you.

⅛ teaspoon saffron threads
2 cups vegetable broth
1 cup basmati rice
¼ cup peanuts
½ teaspoon ground cumin seed
Salt to taste

Plastic Steamers

Soaking the threads in milk, water, stock, an acid mixture (vinegar, lemon juice), or a liquor (vodka, wine, brandy) for a minimum of 20 minutes before you begin to cook will stimulate the release of flavor, aroma, and their characteristic yellow color. Saffron can also be dry roasted in a skillet to help bring out the flavor.

Fill water reservoir to maximum and turn on machine. Add all ingredients to steamer bowl and steam for 50 to 60 minutes. Season and serve.

Nutrition Facts	
Serving Size 5.964 ounces (169.1g)	
Servings Per Container 4	
Amount Per Serving	
Calories 236 Calories from Fat 58	
	% *Daily Value**
Total Fat 6g	9%
Saturated Fat 1g	5%
Cholesterol 0mg	0%
Sodium 173mg	7%
Total Carbohydrate 38g	13%
Dietary Fiber 3g	12%
Sugars 0g	
Protein 8g	
Vitamin A 0%	Vitamin C 0%
Calcium 2%	Iron 8%

*Percent Daily Values are based on a 2,000 calorie diet. Your daily values may be higher or lower depending on your calorie needs.

Metal Steamers

Soaking the threads in milk, water, stock, an acid mixture (vinegar, lemon juice), or a liquor (vodka, wine, brandy) for a minimum of 20 minutes before you begin to cook will stimulate the release of flavor, aroma, and their characteristic yellow color. Saffron can also be dry roasted in a skillet to help bring out the flavor. Coat rice bowl with nonstick spray. Add all ingredients and 1½ cups additional water to bowl and start machine. Season and serve.

Serves 4

Brown Rice Pudding

This is the perfect solution to leftover brown rice.

1 cup short-grain brown rice, cooked
1 cup vanilla soy milk
½ cup raisins or currents
¼ cup sliced almonds
1 egg, lightly whipped
1 tablespoon honey
Salt to taste

Plastic Steamers
Fill water reservoir to maximum and turn on machine. Add all ingredients and steam for 20 minutes. If you are reheating leftover rice pudding, be sure to add a little more soy milk, as it tends to dry out while sitting in the refrigerator.

Metal Steamers
Coat rice bowl with nonstick spray. Add all ingredients plus ½ cup additional water. Cook until all liquid is absorbed. If you are reheating leftover rice pudding, be sure to add a little more soy milk, as it tends to dry out while sitting in the refrigerator.

Serves 4

Nutrition Facts	
Serving Size 5.475 ounces (155.2g)	
Servings Per Container 4	
Amount Per Serving	
Calories 225 Calories from Fat 56	
	% *Daily Value**
Total Fat 6g	9%
Saturated Fat 1g	5%
Cholesterol 53mg	18%
Sodium 52mg	2%
Total Carbohydrate 38g	13%
Dietary Fiber 3g	12%
Sugars 4g	
Protein 6g	
Vitamin A 14%	Vitamin C 2%
Calcium 11%	Iron 10%

*Percent Daily Values are based on a 2,000 calorie diet. Your daily values may be higher or lower depending on your calorie needs.

Brown Rice Crust

This rice crust variation is a great shell for leftover grain dishes.

2 cups medium-grain rice (well cooked)
¼ cup parmesan cheese, grated
1 egg, lightly beaten
Salt to taste

Mix ingredients together. Coat pie pan with nonstick spray and press rice mixture into plate. Bake at 350° for 10 minutes or until golden brown. This is a good shell for quiche or casseroles.

Makes two shells

Nutrition Facts	
Serving Size 8.201 ounces (232.5g)	
Servings Per Container 2	

Amount Per Serving	
Calories 312 Calories from Fat 71	

	% *Daily Value**
Total Fat 8g	12%
Saturated Fat 3g	15%
Cholesterol 116mg	39%
Sodium 266mg	11%
Total Carbohydrate 47g	16%
Dietary Fiber 3g	12%
Sugars 0g	
Protein 13g	

Vitamin A 7%	Vitamin C 0%
Calcium 20%	Iron 8%

*Percent Daily Values are based on a 2,000 calorie diet. Your daily values may be higher or lower depending on your calorie needs.

Aromatic Spiced Rice

So exotic, yet so simple—and a real crowd-pleaser.

2 cups vegetable stock
2 cups brown basmati rice
⅓ cup shelled pistachio nuts
2 teaspoons garam masala (Indian spice mix)

Plastic Steamers

Fill water reservoir to maximum and turn on machine. Steam all ingredients together for 50 to 60 minutes.

Metal Steamers

Coat rice bowl with nonstick spray. Steam all ingredients together with 3 cups of additional water. Let steam on warm for 5 additional minutes.

Serves 8

Nutrition Facts

Serving Size 5.141 ounces (145.8g)
Servings Per Container 8

Amount Per Serving

Calories 234   Calories from Fat 55

	% Daily Value*
Total Fat 6g	9%
Saturated Fat 1g	5%
Cholesterol 0mg	0%
Sodium 295mg	12%
Total Carbohydrate 38g	13%
Dietary Fiber 4g	16%
Sugars 1g	
Protein 7g	

Vitamin A 0%	Vitamin C 0%
Calcium 1%	Iron 6%

*Percent Daily Values are based on a 2,000 calorie diet. Your daily values may be higher or lower depending on your calorie needs.

If you suffer from gluten-sensitive enteropathy, avoid these ingredients:

Almond milk sweetened with
 barley malt
Amaranth*
Barley, barley malt, malt
 flavoring
Brown rice syrup made with
 barley malt enzyme
Buckwheat
Bulgur
Couscous
Distilled white vinegar
Enriched wheat flour, flour
Farina
Gluten, vital gluten
Graham flour
Millet*

Oat groats, rolled oats, oat
 bran
Quinoa*
Rye
Semolina
Soy milk sweetened with
 barley malt or containing
 pearl barley
Spelt*
Teff*
Triticale
Wheat berries, cracked
 wheat, rolled wheat,
 wheat farina
Wheat germ or bran

*May be suitable but more information is needed before these grains can be recommended.

CHAPTER 14

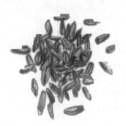

Rye (*Secale cereale*)

Known for its remarkably creamy texture.

Rye originated in southwest Asia. It was domesticated later than wheat, barley, and oats—in about the fourth century B.C. Cultivated rye is said to have originated from wild species that occurred as weeds among wheat and barley crops. Rye was introduced simultaneously and independently at many localities in Central Asia and Asia Minor. It was brought to America by Dutch settlers.

What Is Rye?

Rye is a true grain, being a member of the grass family, Gramineae. It is a vigorous and hardy plant that is similar to wheat and barley. Like wheat, rye does not have a hull. When rye is crossed with wheat, the result is a grain called triticale (see chapter 17).

Nutrition and Rye

Rye is similar in nutrient content to wheat. It does, however, have a better amino acid balance, containing more of the amino acid lysine. Rye is also a good source of B vitamins, especially thiamin and niacin.

One cup of cooked rye berries contains 25% of a day's requirement of magnesium and almost 20% of the required copper and zinc. Rye is also a good source of iron. However, like wheat and triticale, rye also contains phytic acid, which binds some of the minerals in the grain, making them unavailable for absorption. By including a vitamin C source with the meal, much of these minerals will be freed for absorption.

Since rye contains gluten it is not suitable for individuals who are gluten intolerant (celiac disease).

Health and Rye

Cancer Prevention

Like many cereal grains, rye contains phytic acid, saponins, insoluble fiber, and phytoestrogens, all of which appear to decrease the incidences of certain cancers. Rye is also a good source of the flavonoid rutin, vitamin E, and selenium. These compounds are antioxidants that also may protect against cancer.

High Cholesterol

Vitamin E and other antioxidants found in rye may help to protect the heart arteries against the formation of plaque.

How to Buy Rye

Rye flour is available in some supermarkets, but other rye products are usually available only in health food stores and through the mail order companies listed in the back of this book.

Rye Flour

Whole rye flour is made by milling the rye berry. It contains all of the bran and germ. Rye flour is low in gluten and so must be mixed with higher gluten flours for yeast-leavened bread.

Rye Berries

Rye berries are the whole grain kernels. They contain all of the bran and the germ. Rye berries can be used as a breakfast cereal or treated like rice and used in pilafs and casseroles or sprinkled on salads. Presoaking overnight or for a few hours during the day will shorten cooking time.

Rolled Rye

Rolled rye is made by cutting the whole groat into slices, steaming the pieces, and then rolling them flat to form flakes. Rolled rye is sweeter than oatmeal and can be substituted for oatmeal in any recipe.

Cracked Rye

Cracked rye is made by cutting rye kernels to produce a coarse meal. Cracked rye makes a creamy, sweet porridge.

How to Use Rye

Rye berries can be substituted for wheat or rice in most recipes. Rye has a sweeter taste than wheat and is chewier than rice. Use rye berries in pilafs, stuffings, and as an addition to your homemade bread. Cracked rye makes wonderful porridge and pilaf. Substitute rolled rye for rolled oats in breakfast cereal.

Rye products should be stored in an airtight container and kept in a cool, dark place.

Recipes

Basic Cooking Instructions

Rye berries are very hard and will cook faster if presoaked.

1 cup rye berries
1 cup water, juice, or broth
Salt to taste

Soaking instructions: Place rye in steamer bowl and add liquid. Let soak overnight or during the day in the refrigerator.

Plastic Steamers
Fill water reservoir to maximum and turn on machine. Steam for about 50 to 60 minutes. Season and serve. If rye was not pre-soaked, steam for 90 minutes.

Metal Steamers
Coat rice bowl with nonstick spray. Add an additional 1½ cups of water to bowl and cook until machine turns off. Season and let steam for 10 minutes on warm setting. If the rye was not presoaked, add an additional 3 cups of water to the rice bowl before cooking.

Serves 4

Nutrition Facts	
Serving Size 1.490 ounces (42.25g)	
Servings Per Container 4	
Amount Per Serving	
Calories 142 Calories from Fat 9	
	% *Daily Value**
Total Fat 1g	2%
Saturated Fat 0g	0%
Cholesterol 0mg	0%
Sodium 3mg	0%
Total Carbohydrate 30g	10%
Dietary Fiber 2g	8%
Sugars 0g	
Protein 6g	
Vitamin A 0%	Vitamin C 0%
Calcium 1%	Iron 6%

*Percent Daily Values are based on a 2,000 calorie diet. Your daily values may be higher or lower depending on your calorie needs.

Breakfast Rye

An unbelievably creamy cereal. This is a tasty morning dish that keeps you going all morning long. Serve hot and drizzle with milk and honey.

1 cup water
1 cup rolled rye
1 tablespoon blackstrap molasses, honey, or maple syrup
Salt to taste
4 tablespoons date sugar

Plastic Steamer
Fill water reservoir to minimum and turn on machine. Cook all ingredients together for 20 minutes. Season, top each serving with 1 tablespoon date sugar, and serve with milk or juice.

Metal Steamer
Coat rice bowl with nonstick spray. Cook ingredients plus an additional ¼ cup of water. Season and steam on warm for 2 minutes before serving with date sugar and milk or juice.

Serves 4

Nutrition Facts		
Serving Size 1.314 ounces (37.25g)		
Servings Per Container 4		
Amount Per Serving		
Calories 113 Calories from Fat 5		
		% *Daily Value**
Total Fat 1g		2%
Saturated Fat 0g		0%
Cholesterol 0mg		0%
Sodium 6mg		0%
Total Carbohydrate 26g		9%
Dietary Fiber 2g		8%
Sugars 9g		
Protein 3g		
Vitamin A 0%	Vitamin C 0%	
Calcium 4%	Iron 8%	

*Percent Daily Values are based on a 2,000 calorie diet. Your daily values may be higher or lower depending on your calorie needs.

Rye Pilaf

We like to make this with celery and carrot juice fresh from our juicers.

½ cup rye berries, presoaked
½ cup Kamut or spelt, presoaked
1 cup vegetable juice or lowfat chicken broth
1 cup chopped onions
½ tablespoon tamari
½ tablespoon thyme
2 tablespoons parsley, chopped
Salt to taste

Plastic Steamers
Fill water reservoir to maximum and turn on machine. Cook all ingredients together for 60 minutes. Season and serve.

Metal Steamers
Coat rice bowl with nonstick spray. Cook all ingredients plus 1½ cups additional water. Season and steam on warm for 5 minutes before serving.

Serves 4

Nutrition Facts
Serving Size 11.96 ounces (339.0g)
Servings Per Container 4

Amount Per Serving	
Calories 1075 Calories from Fat 6	

	% Daily Value*
Total Fat 1g	2%
Saturated Fat 0g	0%
Cholesterol 0mg	0%
Sodium 56mg	2%
Total Carbohydrate 18g	6%
Dietary Fiber 2g	8%
Sugars 1g	
Protein 4g	

Vitamin A 1%	Vitamin C 7%
Calcium 10%	Iron 5%

*Percent Daily Values are based on a 2,000 calorie diet. Your daily values may be higher or lower depending on your calorie needs.

Vegetable Rye Salad

The combination of cooked grain and raw vegetables makes this salad especially interesting.

1 cup water
1 cup cracked rye
1 clove garlic, minced
1 cup fresh, sliced tomatoes
¼ cup sliced green onions
1 tablespoon chopped fresh parsley or cilantro
¼ teaspoon basil, dried
Salt to taste

Plastic Steamers
Fill water reservoir to maximum and turn on machine. Add water, rye, garlic, and basil to rice bowl and steam for 15 to 20 minutes. Combine with the remaining ingredients and serve.

Metal Steamers
Coat rice bowl with nonstick spray. Add water, rye, garlic, and basil to rice bowl with an additional ½ cup of water. When steamer switches to warm, add remaining ingredients and serve.

Serves 4

Nutrition Facts	
Serving Size 3.526 ounces (99.96g)	
Servings Per Container 4	

Amount Per Serving	
Calories 155 Calories from Fat 11	

	% *Daily Value**
Total Fat 1g	2%
Saturated Fat 0g	0%
Cholesterol 0mg	0%
Sodium 8mg	0%
Total Carbohydrate 32g	11%
Dietary Fiber 3g	12%
Sugars 0g	
Protein 7g	

Vitamin A 4%	Vitamin C 20%
Calcium 2%	Iron 8%

*Percent Daily Values are based on a 2,000 calorie diet. Your daily values may be higher or lower depending on your calorie needs.

Rye Pudding with Strawberry Sauce

Much creamier than rice pudding, this is sure to become a family favorite. This recipe works best in a plastic steamer.

1 cup cooked cracked rye
¾ cup vanilla soy milk
3 tablespoons honey
1 teaspoon vanilla extract
¼ teaspoon nutmeg
Salt to taste
1 egg, slightly beaten

Strawberry Sauce

1 cup fresh or frozen, unsweetened strawberries
2 tablespoons honey

Process till smooth in blender.

Add rye and milk to rice bowl and steam until milk is absorbed, about 5 to 10 minutes. Stir in honey, vanilla, nutmeg, and salt. Remove rice bowl from steamer and when mixture is lukewarm, add egg. Return bowl to steamer and cook for 20 minutes. Serve with Strawberry Sauce.

Serves 4

Nutrition Facts	
Serving Size 5.088 ounces (144.2g)	
Servings Per Container 4	
Amount Per Serving	
Calories 214 Calories from Fat 26	
	% *Daily Value**
Total Fat 3g	5%
Saturated Fat 1g	5%
Cholesterol 53mg	18%
Sodium 41mg	2%
Total Carbohydrate 43g	14%
Dietary Fiber 2g	8%
Sugars 23g	
Protein 6g	
Vitamin A 11%	Vitamin C 35%
Calcium 7%	Iron 7%

*Percent Daily Values are based on a 2,000 calorie diet. Your daily values may be higher or lower depending on your calorie needs.

Rye and Rice

1 cup lowfat chicken or vegetable broth
½ cup rye berries, presoaked
½ cup short-grain brown rice
¼ cup chopped green onions
¼ cup raisins
Salt to taste
15-ounce can garbanzo beans (chick peas), drained (optional)

Plastic Steamers
Fill water reservoir to maximum and turn on machine. Add all ingredients to rice bowl and steam for 60 minutes. Season and serve.

Metal Steamers
Coat rice bowl with nonstick spray. Add ingredients with an additional 1½ cups water and cook until machine turns off. Let steam on warm for 10 minutes. Season and serve.

Serves 4

Nutrition Facts	
Serving Size 3.000 ounces (85.06g)	
Servings Per Container 4	
Amount Per Serving	
Calories 189 Calories from Fat 12	
	% *Daily Value**
Total Fat 1g	2%
Saturated Fat 0g	0%
Cholesterol 0mg	0%
Sodium 100mg	4%
Total Carbohydrate 40g	13%
Dietary Fiber 2g	8%
Sugars 6g	
Protein 6g	
Vitamin A 0%	Vitamin C 0%
Calcium 2%	Iron 6%

*Percent Daily Values are based on a 2,000 calorie diet. Your daily values may be higher or lower depending on your calorie needs.

Peaches and Rye

1 cup water
1 cup rolled rye flakes
1 cup canned peaches, drained
1 tablespoon honey
1 cup lowfat vanilla soy milk
Salt to taste

Plastic Steamers

Fill reservoir with minimum amount of water. Add water and rye to rice bowl and steam for 20 minutes. Season and top cooked rye with peaches and honey. Surround with a moat of soy milk.

Metal Steamers

Coat rice bowl with nonstick spray. Add water and rye with an additional ¼ cup of water and cook. Season and steam on warm for 2 to 5 minutes. Top cooked rye with peaches and honey. Surround with a moat of soy milk.

Nutrition Facts	
Serving Size 5.295 ounces (150.1g)	
Servings Per Container 4	
Amount Per Serving	
Calories 158 Calories from Fat 16	
	% *Daily Value**
Total Fat 2g	3%
Saturated Fat 0g	0%
Cholesterol 0mg	0%
Sodium 35mg	1%
Total Carbohydrate 33g	11%
Dietary Fiber 2g	8%
Sugars 4g	
Protein 5g	
Vitamin A 14%	Vitamin C 7%
Calcium 8%	Iron 7%

*Percent Daily Values are based on a 2,000 calorie diet. Your daily values may be higher or lower depending on your calorie needs.

CHAPTER 15

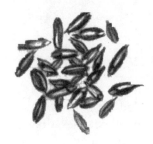

Spelt *(Triticum aestivum spelta)*

Cooked kernels have a sweet, nutty taste and ricelike texture.

Spelt is at least fifteen hundred years older than our modern wheat. It was a common grain in Biblical times and is mentioned several times in the Bible. In the book of Exodus, Moses caused hail to destroy the crops ". . . but the spelt and rye were not smitten." Folklore has it that back in the fifteenth century, a young Saint Hildegard used this grain to heal the sick. She claimed to have a vision from God who told her to feed her charges spelt.

In Germany, spelt is called *dinkle*. After losing favor to the higher yielding modern wheat, dinkle is again becoming popular in Germany, where farmers are having a hard time keeping up with demand.

What Is Spelt?

Spelt is a primitive form of grain that is related to wheat. However, modern wheat is a hybrid, and spelt is not. Its proponents believe this is why spelt is tolerated better by people who suffer from allergies.

Physically, spelt looks like wheat but is softer, larger, and redder in color.

Nutrition and Spelt

Spelt is very similar to its close relative wheat. It is an excellent source of protein, of the minerals magnesium, zinc, copper, and iron, and of the B vitamins thiamin and riboflavin.

Because spelt contains high amounts of gluten, it should be totally avoided by those who suffer from celiac disease or gluten intolerance.

Health and Spelt

Since spelt is a specialty grain that has only recently begun growing in popularity, no research has been done specifically on spelt. However, since spelt is very similar to wheat, many of the health benefits of wheat can be extrapolated to spelt.

Cancer Prevention

Spelt is a source of insoluble fiber, which has been associated with a decreased risk of colon and rectal cancer.

Constipation

Fiber increases the bulk of the feces and relieves constipation. A high-fiber diet also decreases the risk of problems associated with constipation: hemorrhoids and diverticular disease.

Wheat Allergies

If you have a mild allergy to wheat, you might consider adding spelt to your diet. Since spelt contains many of the same proteins as wheat, if you have a severe wheat allergy, try spelt only under your physician's supervision.

How to Buy Spelt

Spelt is a specialty grain and is not yet commonly available in supermarkets. Spelt can be bought at some health food stores or ordered through the mail order sources in the back of the book.

Spelt Berries

Spelt berries are the whole kernel with all of the bran and germ intact. They have a sweet, nutty flavor and a texture similar to rice. Use spelt berries in casseroles, pilafs, and sprinkled on salads or in any recipe that calls for rice.

Spelt Flour

Spelt flour is made from whole grain spelt. It is higher in gluten than other grains and makes a wonderful alternative to wheat flour. Spelt flour can be substituted equally for wheat flour.

Rolled Spelt

Rolled spelt or spelt flakes are groats which have been cut into slices, steamed, and then rolled into thick flakes. Rolled spelt makes a wonderful breakfast cereal and can be substituted for rolled oats or wheat in any recipe.

How to Use Spelt

Spelt berries can be substituted for wheat, rye, or rice in most recipes. It is softer than wheat and chewier than rice. Use spelt berries in pilafs, stuffings, and as an addition to homemade bread. Rolled spelt makes a nice change from rolled oats as a breakfast cereal.

Spelt products should be stored in an airtight container and kept in a cool, dark place.

Recipes

Basic Cooking Instructions

Steamed spelt berries are our favorite whole grain berries. They steam up larger and plumper than wheat and have a smooth exterior. We love to sprinkle them on salads, where they add to the eye appeal.

Spelt berries are very hard and will cook faster if pre-soaked.

1 cup spelt berries
1 cup water, juice, or broth
Salt to taste

Soaking instructions: Place spelt into rice bowl and add liquid. Let soak overnight or during the day in refrigerator. Drain grains and add back 1 cup water or replace with another liquid.

Plastic Steamers
Fill water reservoir to maximum and turn on machine. Steam for about 50 to 60 minutes. Season and serve. If spelt was not pre-soaked, steam for 90 minutes.

Metal Steamers
Add an additional 1½ cup of water to steamer bowl and cook until machine turns off. Season and let steam for 5 minutes on warm setting. If spelt was not presoaked, add an additional 3 cups of water to rice bowl before cooking.

Serves 4

Nutrition Facts	
Serving Size 1.675 ounces (47.50g)	
Servings Per Container 4	
Amount Per Serving	
Calories 184 Calories from Fat 14	
	% *Daily Value**
Total Fat 2g	3%
Saturated Fat 0g	0%
Cholesterol 0mg	0%
Sodium 0mg	0%
Total Carbohydrate 35g	12%
Dietary Fiber 0g	0%
Sugars 0g	
Protein 6g	
Vitamin A -% Vitamin C -%	
Calcium -% Iron 2%	

*Percent Daily Values are based on a 2,000 calorie diet. Your daily values may be higher or lower depending on your calorie needs.

Breakfast Spelt

A wonderful alternative to oatmeal in the morning. The apple juice and dates add a fragrant, natural sweetness that is not overwhelming.

1 cup rolled spelt
1 cup apple juice
¼ cup chopped dates
1 teaspoon cinnamon
Salt to taste
2 cups of 1% fat milk or soy milk

Plastic Steamers
Fill reservoir to minimum with water and turn on machine. Add all ingredients except milk to rice bowl and steam for 20 minutes. Season, then place ½ cup of cereal in serving bowl and add milk or soy milk.

Metal Steamers
Coat rice bowl with nonstick spray. Add all ingredients except milk to rice bowl and turn on machine. After machine turns off, season and let steam for 1 or 2 minutes on warm. Place ½ cup of cereal in serving bowl and add milk or soy milk.

Serves 4

Nutrition Facts	
Serving Size 7.988 ounces (226.4g)	
Servings Per Container 4	
Amount Per Serving	
Calories 229 Calories from Fat 22	
	% *Daily Value**
Total Fat 2g	3%
Saturated Fat 1g	5%
Cholesterol 5mg	2%
Sodium 64mg	3%
Total Carbohydrate 44g	15%
Dietary Fiber 1g	4%
Sugars 13g	
Protein 8g	
Vitamin A 7%	Vitamin C 45%
Calcium 16%	Iron 5%

*Percent Daily Values are based on a 2,000 calorie diet. Your daily values may be higher or lower depending on your calorie needs.

Spelt Pilaf

The spelt grain's resiliency gives a bite that is perfect as a pilaf.

1 cup of lowfat chicken broth
½ cup of presoaked spelt
½ cup of medium-grain brown rice
¼ cup finely chopped parsley
¼ cup finely chopped dates
⅛ cup finely chopped green onions
Salt to taste

Plastic Steamers
Fill reservoir to minimum with water and turn on machine. Add ingredients to rice bowl and steam for 50 to 60 minutes. Season and serve.

Metal Steamers
Coat rice bowl with nonstick spray. Add ingredients to rice bowl with an additional 1 cup of water and turn on machine. After machine turns off, season and let steam for 5 minutes on warm.

Serves 4

Nutrition Facts	
Serving Size 4.603 ounces (130.5g)	
Servings Per Container 4	
Amount Per Serving	
Calories 244 Calories from Fat 19	
	% *Daily Value**
Total Fat 2g	3%
Saturated Fat 0g	0%
Cholesterol 0mg	0%
Sodium 197mg	8%
Total Carbohydrate 49g	16%
Dietary Fiber 2g	8%
Sugars 7g	
Protein 7g	
Vitamin A 2%	Vitamin C 6%
Calcium 1%	Iron 6%

*Percent Daily Values are based on a 2,000 calorie diet. Your daily values may be higher or lower depending on your calorie needs.

Dilled Spelt Salad

Fresh dill and lemon juice give this cold salad zip.

1 cup lowfat chicken or vegetable broth
1 cup spelt berries, presoaked
1 cup julienne snow peas
1 red pepper, chopped
2 tablespoons fresh, chopped dill leaves
1 tablespoon lemon juice
1 tablespoon olive or canola oil
Salt to taste

Plastic Steamers
Fill water reservoir to maximum and turn on machine. Add presoaked grain and broth and steam for about 50 to 60 minutes. Combine cooked grain in a large bowl with raw vegetables, oil, and seasonings.

Metal Steamers
Coat rice bowl with nonstick spray. Add an additional 1½ cups of water to presoaked spelt and broth, and cook until machine turns off. Let steam for 5 minutes on warm setting. Combine cooked grain in a large bowl with raw vegetables, oil, and seasonings.

Serves 4

Nutrition Facts	
Serving Size 7.079 ounces (200.7g)	
Servings Per Container 4	
Amount Per Serving	
Calories 295 Calories from Fat 53	
	% *Daily Value**
Total Fat 6g	9%
Saturated Fat 1g	5%
Cholesterol 0mg	0%
Sodium 199mg	8%
Total Carbohydrate 49g	16%
Dietary Fiber 2g	8%
Sugars 0g	
Protein 11g	
Vitamin A 2%	Vitamin C 85%
Calcium 4%	Iron 11%

*Percent Daily Values are based on a 2,000 calorie diet. Your daily values may be higher or lower depending on your calorie needs.

Country Breakfast Spelt

Prunes are a delicious sweetener in this cereal. A great way to keep regular.

1 cup spelt berries, presoaked
1 cup water or fruit juice
½ cup chopped prunes (or seedless raisins)
1 teaspoon cinnamon
Salt to taste

Plastic Steamers
Fill reservoir to minimum with water and turn on machine. Add ingredients to rice bowl and steam for 50 to 60 minutes. Season and serve.

Metal Steamers
Coat rice bowl with nonstick spray. Add ingredients to rice bowl with an additional 1 cup of water and turn on machine. After machine turns off, season and let steam for 5 minutes on warm.

Serves 4

Nutrition Facts	
Serving Size 2.406 ounces (68.20g)	
Servings Per Container 4	
Amount Per Serving	
Calories 233 Calories from Fat 15	
	% *Daily Value**
Total Fat 2g	3%
Saturated Fat 0g	0%
Cholesterol 0mg	0%
Sodium 1mg	0%
Total Carbohydrate 48g	16%
Dietary Fiber 1g	4%
Sugars 9g	
Protein 7g	
Vitamin A 4%	Vitamin C 1%
Calcium 1%	Iron 6%

*Percent Daily Values are based on a 2,000 calorie diet. Your daily values may be higher or lower depending on your calorie needs.

CHAPTER 16

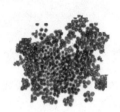

Teff *(Eragrostis tef)*

This tiny grain is dark brown and has a light, nutty flavor.

*T*eff is an Amharic word meaning "lost," which describes what happens to this tiny grain if you drop it. Teff was brought to the United States from Ethiopia by a Peace Corp worker who has since been raising it on his farm.

What Is Teff?

Teff is the seed of a drought-resistant plant. It is a tiny seed, smaller even than amaranth. One hundred fifty grains of teff weigh the same as one grain of wheat. It is mild in flavor, with a slightly sweet molasseslike taste. It is from the genus *Eragrostis*, which contains no other plants eaten for food.

Teff is used in Ethiopia to make the staple Ethiopian flat bread *injera*. There are three strains of teff. Reddish teff is usually sold only to Ethiopian restaurants. Brown teff is available from Arrowhead Mills. Ivory teff is available directly from the grower.

Nutrition and Teff

Teff is not related to wheat so it can be tolerated by those with wheat allergies. Not enough is known about the biochemical composition of teff as yet to recommend it to those who are gluten intolerant (celiac disease). Until further analysis and studies are performed, teff should be totally avoided by those who are gluten intolerant.

This grain is so small it cannot be refined, so all teff is whole grain. All of the bran and germ are intact. This means that teff is mineral and fiber rich. Teff has more calcium than either wheat or barley and is also rich in thiamin and iron. Since teff is so small in diameter, it contains a greater percentage of fiber than most larger grains. Teff is a good source of soluble fiber. Ivory teff, although light in color, is not a refined grain and contains all the same nutrients as its brown and red relatives.

How to Buy Teff

Teff is grown by only one farm in the United States. Brown teff is available directly from the grower and from Arrowhead Mills. Ask for it at your local health food store or order it from the suppliers listed in the back of the book. Ivory teff can be purchased directly from the grower (also listed).

How to Use Teff

Teff is a very small grain that mixes well with a variety of other, larger grains. It can be enjoyed as a porridge, combined with other grains in a pilaf, and used as a stuffing, a topping for appetizers, or a garnish for green salads. Teff is easier to chew if the grain is toasted or soaked before steaming.

Teff should be sealed in a container and stored in a cool, dry place.

Recipes

Basic Cooking Instructions

Teff benefits from dry roasting before steaming. Not only does the roasting develop a wonderful nutty flavor, it makes this tiny seed open up and accept other flavors more readily.

½ to ¾ cup water, juice, or broth
½ cup teff
Salt to taste

Plastic Steamers

Fill reservoir with water and turn on machine. Add ingredients to rice bowl and steam for 20 to 25 minutes. Season and serve.

Metal Steamers

Coat rice bowl with nonstick spray. Add ingredients to rice bowl with an additonal ½ to ¾ cup of water and turn on machine. After machine turns off, season and let steam for 5 minutes on warm.

Serves 4

Nutrition Facts	
Serving Size 1.000 ounces (28.35g)	
Servings Per Container 4	

Amount Per Serving	
Calories 101 Calories from Fat 5	

	% *Daily Value**
Total Fat 1g	2%
Saturated Fat 0g	0%
Cholesterol 0mg	0%
Sodium 5mg	0%
Total Carbohydrate 21g	7%
Dietary Fiber 4g	16%
Sugars 0g	
Protein 4g	

Vitamin A -%	Vitamin C -%
Calcium 0%	Iron 70%

*Percent Daily Values are based on a 2,000 calorie diet. Your daily values may be higher or lower depending on your calorie needs.

Breakfast Teff

A delightful change of pace from the usual porridges or flakes.

1⅜ cups water
½ cup teff
¼ cup dried cranberries, chopped
2 tablespoons molasses
½ teaspoon nutmeg
Salt to taste
Milk or soy milk

Plastic Steamers
Fill reservoir to minimum with water and turn on machine. Add teff, water, cranberries, molasses, and nutmeg to rice bowl. Steam for 20 minutes, season, top with milk, and serve.

Metal Steamers
Coat rice bowl with nonstick spray. Add ingredients to rice bowl with an additional ½ cup of water. After machine turns off, season and let steam for 1 or 2 minutes on warm. Top with milk and serve.

Serves 4

Nutrition Facts	
Serving Size 1.847 ounces (52.38g)	
Servings Per Container 4	
Amount Per Serving	
Calories 132 Calories from Fat 6	
	% *Daily Value**
Total Fat 1g	2%
Saturated Fat 0g	0%
Cholesterol 0mg	0%
Sodium 14mg	1%
Total Carbohydrate 28g	9%
Dietary Fiber 5g	20%
Sugars 4g	
Protein 4g	
Vitamin A 0%	Vitamin C 3%
Calcium 7%	Iron 79%

*Percent Daily Values are based on a 2,000 calorie diet. Your daily values may be higher or lower depending on your calorie needs.

Teff Pilaf

A fast side dish for dinner. Add chopped apple to this pilaf for
a perfect cold picnic dish.

1 cup toasted cooked teff
1 cup cooked short-grain brown rice
2 tablespoons chopped walnuts
2 tablespoons dry white wine
3 tablespoons chopped baby dill

Combine ingredients and warm in steamer for 5 minutes.

Serves 4

Nutrition Facts	
Serving Size 2.618 ounces (74.21g)	
Servings Per Container 4	
Amount Per Serving	
Calories 134 Calories from Fat 26	
	% *Daily Value**
Total Fat 3g	5%
Saturated Fat 0g	0%
Cholesterol 0mg	0%
Sodium 3mg	0%
Total Carbohydrate 22g	7%
Dietary Fiber 3g	12%
Sugars 0g	
Protein 4g	
Vitamin A 0%	Vitamin C 0%
Calcium 1%	Iron 37%

*Percent Daily Values are based on a
2,000 calorie diet. Your daily values
may be higher or lower depending on
your calorie needs.

Teff Caviar Salad

This delicate dish *looks* like caviar and is a great topping for green salads, or for raw or steamed vegetables.

½ cup lowfat chicken or vegetable broth
½ cup teff
3 tablespoons parsley
1 stalk celery, finely chopped
1 tablespoon fresh mint, finely chopped
1 tablespoon currants, chopped
Salt to taste

Plastic Steamers

Fill reservoir to minimum with water and turn on machine. Add ingredients to rice bowl and steam for 20 minutes. Season and serve.

Metal Steamers

Coat rice bowl with nonstick spray. Add ingredients to rice bowl plus an additional 1 cup of water and turn on machine. After machine turns off, season and let steam for 1 or 2 minutes on warm. Season and serve.

Serves 4

Nutrition Facts	
Serving Size 2.215 ounces (62.81g)	
Servings Per Container 4	
Amount Per Serving	
Calories 188 Calories from Fat 66	
	% *Daily Value**
Total Fat 7g	11%
Saturated Fat 1g	5%
Cholesterol 0mg	0%
Sodium 42mg	2%
Total Carbohydrate 27g	9%
Dietary Fiber 4g	16%
Sugars 0g	
Protein 4g	
Vitamin A 0%	Vitamin C 7%
Calcium 1%	Iron 76%

*Percent Daily Values are based on a 2,000 calorie diet. Your daily values may be higher or lower depending on your calorie needs.

Teff Salad

Surprise your friends with this unusual starter. Serve this luscious spread on toast or French bread.

½ cup lowfat chicken broth
½ cup teff
2 cloves fresh garlic, crushed
½ teaspoon fresh ground pepper
¼ cup green olives, finely chopped
1 tablespoon olive oil or olive-flavored water from the can
    (optional)

Plastic Steamers
Mix all ingredients in steamer bowl except olives and cook for 20 minutes. Add olives and, if desired, a splash of olive oil or olive-flavored water and serve.

Metal Steamers
Coat steamer bowl with non-stick spray. Mix all ingredients in bowl except olives. Add an additional ½ cup of water and cook until all water is absorbed. Add olives and, if desired, a splash of olive oil or olive-flavored water and serve.

Nutrition Facts	
Serving Size 3.386 ounces (96.00g)	
Servings Per Container 4	
Amount Per Serving	
Calories 121 Calories from Fat 18	
	% *Daily Value**
Total Fat 2g	3%
Saturated Fat 0g	0%
Cholesterol 0mg	0%
Sodium 42mg	12%
Total Carbohydrate 22g	7%
Dietary Fiber 5g	20%
Sugars 0g	
Protein 5g	
Vitamin A 0%	Vitamin C 1%
Calcium 1%	Iron 72%

*Percent Daily Values are based on a 2,000 calorie diet. Your daily values may be higher or lower depending on your calorie needs.

Harvest Teff

This recipe also works well with 1 part teff to 1 part quinoa.

½ cup water
2 cups chopped, unpeeled apples
½ cup teff
1 cup green onions, chopped
1 tablespoon sesame seeds
Salt to taste

Plastic Steamers

Fill reservoir to minimum with water and turn on machine. Add ingredients to rice bowl and steam for 20 minutes. Season and serve.

Metal Steamers

Coat rice bowl with nonstick spray. Add ingredients plus an additional ½ cup of water to rice bowl and turn on machine. After machine turns off, season and let steam for 1 or 2 minutes on warm. Season and serve.

Serves 4

Nutrition Facts	
Serving Size 2.608 ounces (73.93g)	
Servings Per Container 4	
Amount Per Serving	
Calories 97 Calories from Fat 14	
	% *Daily Value**
Total Fat 2g	3%
Saturated Fat 0g	0%
Cholesterol 0mg	0%
Sodium 3mg	0%
Total Carbohydrate 19g	6%
Dietary Fiber 4g	16%
Sugars 7g	
Protein 2g	
Vitamin A 1%	Vitamin C 7%
Calcium 2%	Iron 37%

*Percent Daily Values are based on a 2,000 calorie diet. Your daily values may be higher or lower depending on your calorie needs.

Thyme Teff

Simple and delicious, this can be a spread for crackers or a layer in a casserole. It's wonderful on its own as well.

½ cup vegetable broth
1 cup teff
2 tablespoons fresh thyme, chopped or 2 teaspoons dried
Salt to taste

Plastic Steamers
Fill reservoir to minimum with water and turn on machine. Add ingredients to rice bowl and steam for 20 minutes. Season and serve.

Metal Steamers
Coat rice bowl with nonstick spray. Add ingredients to rice bowl plus an additional ½ cup of water and turn on machine. After machine turns off, season and let steam for 1 or 2 minutes on warm. Season and serve.

Serves 4

Nutrition Facts	
Serving Size 5.316 ounces (150.7g)	
Servings Per Container 4	
Amount Per Serving	
Calories 122 Calories from Fat 11	
	% *Daily Value**
Total Fat 1g	2%
Saturated Fat 0g	0%
Cholesterol 0mg	0%
Sodium 42mg	16%
Total Carbohydrate 21g	7%
Dietary Fiber 4g	16%
Sugars 0g	
Protein 6g	
Vitamin A 0%	Vitamin C 0%
Calcium 1%	Iron 74%

*Percent Daily Values are based on a 2,000 calorie diet. Your daily values may be higher or lower depending on your calorie needs.

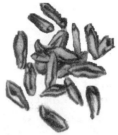

CHAPTER 17

Triticale (*Triticale heraploide*)

Triticale berries look like large plump wheat berries.

*P*ronounced *trit-uh-cah-lee*. Botanists first crossbred wheat and rye in 1876. This yielded a plant that could not produce seeds. In 1937, scientists discovered that treating seedlings of wheat–rye crosses with a chemical called colchicine made the plants fertile. By the 1950s many countries had triticale breeding programs. Triticale may become an important food in areas not suited for wheat production. Some varieties can grow in cold climates and in sandy or acid soils. Others resist disease-causing rust fungi better than wheat.

What Is Triticale?

Triticale is a true cereal grain. It is a hybrid obtained from a cross between wheat and rye that is hardier and more nutritious than either parent. It has a sweet, nutty flavor.

Nutrition and Triticale

Triticale is more nutritous than either parent grain. It is an excellent source of protein. One cup of cooked triticale groats provides over a quarter of the protein needed for a day. Like its parent grains, triticale is low in lysine and methionine. But also like its parents, it is an excellent source of minerals, including magnesium, iron, copper, and zinc; of B vitamins, including thiamin, riboflavin, niacin, folate, and pyridoxine; and of the fat-soluble vitamin E.

Because triticale is a cross between wheat and rye, it is not suitable for individuals who suffer from wheat or rye allergies or for those who are gluten intolerant.

Health and Triticale

Cancer Prevention

Triticale has most of the postulated cancer-preventing substances found in wheat including phytic acid, insoluble fiber, selenium, and phytosterols.

Vegetarians

Triticale provides more protein than most grains, so it is a good choice for individuals who do not eat meat or animal products. It is especially important during times of growth such as childhood, adolescence, pregnancy, and lactation. Triticale is also a good source of iron; but because the phytic acid in it may bind much of the iron, a vitamin C source must be eaten with the cereal to counter this. Foods that contain vitamin C can be found in chapter 5.

How to Buy Triticale

Triticale is available in only a few forms. You can purchase a home mill to grind your own triticale at some health food stores.

Triticale Berries

Triticale berries are the whole uncrushed grains that have been dehulled. They are chewy and nutritious when cooked. For faster steaming, presoak overnight or during the day for 4 to 6 hours.

Triticale Meal

Triticale meal is made by stone grinding the whole berries to produce a farina-like cereal. It makes a good breakfast porridge.

Rolled Triticale

Rolled triticale, or triticale flakes, is made by cutting triticale berries into slices and then rolling the slices to form flakes. These flakes make an excellent breakfast cereal and can be substituted for oat flakes in any recipe.

How to Use Triticale

Rolled triticale and triticale meal can be used as breakfast cereals. Triticale berries can be substituted for rice and used to make stuffings and pilafs or sprinkled on salads.

Triticale should be stored in a sealed container and kept in a cool, dark place. It will keep for up to nine months.

Recipes

Basic Cooking Instructions

Triticale berries, like wheat and rye berries, are very hard. The cooking time can be greatly reduced by presoaking.

1 cup triticale berries
1 cup water, juice, or broth
Salt to taste

To presoak: Add berries and cooking liquid to rice bowl and let sit overnight or during the day in refrigerator.

Plastic Steamers

Fill reservoir to maximum with water and turn on machine. Add water and grain to rice bowl and steam for 50 to 60 minutes. If grain was not presoaked, refill reservoir with water and steam for an additional 30 minutes. Season and serve.

Metal Steamers

Coat rice bowl with nonstick spray. Add ingredients to rice bowl with an additional 1 cup of water and turn on machine. After machine turns off, season and let steam for 1 or 2 minutes on warm. If grain was not presoaked, add an additional 1 cup of water and cook until machine turns off; season and let grain steam for 5 minutes before serving.

Serves 4

Nutrition Facts	
Serving Size 1.693 ounces (48.00g)	
Servings Per Container 4	

Amount Per Serving	
Calories 162 Calories from Fat 9	

	% Daily Value*
Total Fat 1g	2%
Saturated Fat 0g	0%
Cholesterol 0mg	0%
Sodium 2mg	0%
Total Carbohydrate 35g	12%
Dietary Fiber 0g	0%
Sugars 0g	
Protein 6g	

Vitamin A -%	Vitamin C 0%
Calcium 1%	Iron 6%

*Percent Daily Values are based on a 2,000 calorie diet. Your daily values may be higher or lower depending on your calorie needs.

Breakfast Triticale

This recipe will give you lots of protein to keep you going throughout the morning. It also is very fiber rich.

1 cup 1% fat milk or soy milk
½ cup rolled triticale
½ cup rolled rye
2 tablespoons honey
1 tablespoon oat bran
1 tablespoon psyllium seed or flaxseed
Salt to taste

Plastic Steamers
Fill reservoir to minimum with water and turn on machine. Add ingredients to rice bowl and steam for 20 minutes. Season, add ½ cup additional milk, and serve.

Metal Steamers
Coat rice bowl with nonstick spray. Add ingredients with an additional ½ cup water and turn on machine. After machine turns off, season and let steam for 1 or 2 minutes on warm. Add ½ cup additional milk to cereal and serve.

Serves 4

Nutrition Facts	
Serving Size 5.646 ounces (160.1g)	
Servings Per Container 4	
Amount Per Serving	
Calories 180 Calories from Fat 28	
	% Daily Value*
Total Fat 3g	5%
Saturated Fat 1g	5%
Cholesterol 5mg	2%
Sodium 66mg	3%
Total Carbohydrate 33g	11%
Dietary Fiber 1g	4%
Sugars 14g	
Protein 8g	
Vitamin A 7%	Vitamin C 2%
Calcium 16%	Iron 6%

*Percent Daily Values are based on a 2,000 calorie diet. Your daily values may be higher or lower depending on your calorie needs.

Triticale Pilaf

Italian seasonings such as garlic salt, oregano, and basil are a nice complement to this grain's natural flavors.

1 cup tomato juice
½ cup presoaked triticale berries
½ cup brown rice
2 teaspoons Italian seasoning
2 teaspoons minced garlic
1 teaspoon olive oil
¼ teaspoon pepper
Salt to taste

Plastic Steamers
Fill reservoir to minimum with water and turn on machine. Add ingredients to rice bowl and steam for 60 minutes. Season and serve.

Metal Steamers
Coat rice bowl with nonstick spray. Add ingredients with an additional 1 cup water and turn on machine. After machine turns off, season and let steam for 1 or 2 minutes on warm. Season and serve.

Serves 4

Nutrition Facts	
Serving Size 3.907 ounces (110.8g)	
Servings Per Container 4	
Amount Per Serving	
Calories 188 Calories from Fat 21	
	% *Daily Value**
Total Fat 2g	3%
Saturated Fat 0g	0%
Cholesterol 0mg	0%
Sodium 9mg	0%
Total Carbohydrate 38g	13%
Dietary Fiber 1g	4%
Sugars 2g	
Protein 5g	
Vitamin A 3%	Vitamin C 19%
Calcium 2%	Iron 8%

*Percent Daily Values are based on a 2,000 calorie diet. Your daily values may be higher or lower depending on your calorie needs.

Triticale and Fruit

Hearty grains mixed with fruits make a delightful lunchtime meal.

1 cup triticale berries, presoaked
1 cup water or apple juice
1 apple, chopped
¼ cup raisins, chopped
Salt to taste

To presoak: Add berries and cooking liquid to rice bowl and let sit overnight or during the day in refrigerator.

Plastic Steamers

Fill reservoir to maximum with water and turn on machine. Steam for 50 to 60 minutes. If grain was not presoaked, refill reservoir with water and steam for an additional 30 minutes. Season and serve.

Metal Steamers

Coat rice bowl with nonstick spray. Add ingredients to rice bowl with an additional 1 cup of water and turn on machine. After machine turns off, season and let steam for 1 or 2 minutes on warm. If grain was not pre-soaked, add an additional 1 cup of water and cook until machine turns off. Season and serve.

Serves 4

Nutrition Facts	
Serving Size 5.443 ounces (154.3g)	
Servings Per Container 4	

Amount Per Serving	
Calories 238 Calories from Fat 11	

	% *Daily Value**
Total Fat 1g	2%
Saturated Fat 0g	0%
Cholesterol 0mg	0%
Sodium 6mg	0%
Total Carbohydrate 55g	18%
Dietary Fiber 1g	4%
Sugars 10g	
Protein 7g	

Vitamin A 0%	Vitamin C 46%
Calcium 2%	Iron 9%

*Percent Daily Values are based on a 2,000 calorie diet. Your daily values may be higher or lower depending on your calorie needs.

Triticale Salad

The yogurt makes a surprisingly creamy dressing for this salad of many textures.

1 cup water
½ cup triticale berries, presoaked
2 tablespoons spelt or Kamut, presoaked
2 tablespoons short-grain brown rice
2 tablespoons wild rice, presoaked
2 tablespoons quinoa
1 green onion, chopped
½ cup nonfat raspberry yogurt

Plastic Steamers
Fill reservoir to maximum with water and turn on machine. Steam for 50 to 60 minutes. Season and cool. Mix in yogurt and serve.

Metal Steamers
Coat rice bowl with nonstick spray. Add ingredients to rice bowl and turn on machine. After machine turns off, season and let steam for 1 or 2 minutes on warm. If grain was not pre-soaked, add an additional 1 cup of water and cook until machine turns off. Season and cool. Mix in yogurt and serve.

Serves 4

Nutrition Facts	
Serving Size 3.228 ounces (91.50g)	
Servings Per Container 4	
Amount Per Serving	
Calories 207 Calories from Fat 11	
	% *Daily Value**
Total Fat 1g	2%
Saturated Fat 0g	0%
Cholesterol 1mg	0%
Sodium 27mg	1%
Total Carbohydrate 43g	14%
Dietary Fiber 0g	0%
Sugars 0g	
Protein 8g	
Vitamin A 0%	Vitamin C 0%
Calcium 7%	Iron 7%

*Percent Daily Values are based on a 2,000 calorie diet. Your daily values may be higher or lower depending on your calorie needs.

CHAPTER 18

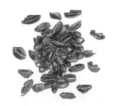

Wheat *(Triticum aestivum)*

This familiar grain comes in a wide variety of forms. The whole grain is a suitable rice alternative.

Wheat is one of the oldest and most important cultivated food plants. Long before the beginnings of agriculture, people gathered wild wheat for food. Several varieties of emmer wheat (*Triticum dicoccum*) have been found in rubbish heaps that date to the end of the Neolithic epoch, a little before the Bronze Age. Scholars believe that about eleven thousand years ago, people in the Middle East took the first steps toward agriculture and that wheat was one of the first plants they grew. In time, these early farmers raised more grain than they needed to feed themselves. People no longer had to wander continuously to search for food. This enabled them to form settlements. Some areas grew enough grain to feed people of other lands, and trade was developed. Villages became thriving cities. in cities, many people did not have to produce their own food and were freed to develop other useful skills. Over time, these changes led to the building of more towns and cities, the expansion of trade, and the development of the great civilizations of ancient Egypt, India, and Mesopotamia.

What Is Wheat?

Wheat is a member of the grass family, Gramineae. Wheat grains are ovoid in shape—rounded at both ends. They are composed of three main parts: the starchy endosperm, the fibrous bran, and the oil-rich germ. Refined wheat products contain only the endosperm of the kernel; they lack the nutrient-rich bran and germ.

There are two main types of wheat: hard and soft. Hard wheat has a higher protein content, around 17%. Because of its high gluten content, hard wheat is used in bread baking. Soft wheat has a lower protein content and is used in cake baking. Durum wheat is a type of hard wheat that is used for making pasta and couscous.

Nutrition and Wheat

Wheat is the staple grain of almost one third of the world's population. The wheat berry contains protein, carbohydrates, both soluble and insoluble fiber, vitamins, and minerals, as well as a number of phytochemicals. It is an excellent source of protein. However, like all true cereals, it contains less of the essential amino acids lysine and methionine than animal products. This means that individuals who eat no animal protein must include lysine-rich foods such as beans and seeds in their diet to balance out the amino acid levels. One cup of rolled wheat will supply 11% of the protein needed for the day. It is a very good source of vitamin E, as well as providing magnesium, iron, zinc, and the B vitamins.

Wheat's main claim to fame, however, is its fiber content. Some of the benefits of fiber are expanded upon below. Since wheat also contains substantial amounts of phytic acid, a compound which binds minerals, a vitamin C source should be included in any meal containing wheat. Vitamin C increases the amount of minerals available from wheat.

Since wheat is an excellent source of gluten, it should be totally avoided by those with gluten intolerance (celiac disease).

Health and Wheat

Brain Functioning

Wheat germ is rich in thiamin. Thiamin is necessary for proper nerve function. In studies, low thiamin levels have been linked to impairment of brain activity.

Cancer

Wheat is a good source of selenium, which is as bioavailable from wheat as the selenium in meat. Along with the other antioxidant vitamins, it has been inversely related to cancer risk in epidemiologic studies. Also a high-fiber diet has been associated with reduced risks of breast, stomach, and prostate cancers.

Colon Cancer Prevention

Studies have shown that the addition of 1.5 ounces of wheat bran each day inhibited DNA synthesis and reduced cell proliferation in the colon. Those are conditions that could lead to cancerous lesions. Researchers believe that the phytic acid in wheat, and especially in wheat bran, may be a potent anti-cancer agent.

Constipation

Wheat bran is one of the most recommended treatments for constipation. It decreases the time it takes for food to travel through the colon. Add 2 tablespoons of wheat bran to your morning cereal or spinkle it on salads or casseroles. Start with 1 tablespoon and gradually work up to 2 tablespoons.

High Cholesterol

When male rats were fed wheat germ, the wheat germ was able to trap cholesterol in the gut, making it unavailable for reabsorption. The researchers felt that the phytosterols in the wheat germ were the agent responsible.

Irritable Bowel Syndrome (IBS)

IBS results in alternating cramps and diarrhea. In one study, 2 tablespoons of bran were all that was necessary to reduce symptoms. However, sometimes IBS is caused by food allergies, and wheat is one of the most common food allergens. If you have IBS, try eliminating all wheat from your diet. Substitute other grains in this book. If the symptoms disappear or are greatly reduced, consider removing wheat permanently from your diet. Rice bran can be substituted for the wheat bran.

Menopausal Symptoms

Hot flashes and other menopausal symptoms are less common among Japanese women than among Western women. Some researchers feel that plant estrogens may be the reason. These phytoestrogens may be able to supplement the decreasing levels of estrogen in the postmenopausal woman. Wheat germ is an especially good source of these compounds.

Osteoporosis

Wheat is a good source of magnesium, which is important for bone metabolism. Researchers have found that animals who are deficient in this trace mineral are at risk for developing severe osteoporosis.

How to Buy Wheat

Wheat comes in a dizzying variety of forms. Always choose whole grain wheat products whenever possible. Most of these products can be purchased in your local supermarket, but some, like whole wheat couscous and farina, may be harder to locate. Try your local health food store or one of the mail order companies listed in the back of the book. Buying grains in bulk is a real money saver and also makes good sense if you only need a small amount of grain.

Bulgur

Bulgur is a product made by partially cooking the wheat kernel, followed by parching and then cracking the grain between rollers. Bulgur can be made from hard red wheat or soft white wheat. Each type has its own special texture and taste. It is a staple grain in southeastern Europe and the Middle East and is becoming increasing popular in this country. Because bulgur is precooked, it requires very little time in the steamer to prepare.

Couscous

Couscous is similar to bulgur. It is made from durum wheat, which is high in protein and gluten. We recommend only whole wheat couscous. This product is made by grinding the whole durum wheat kernel into flour, mixing the flour with water, and forming the result into long strands. The strands are then broken into pieces, steamed, and dried. In the steamer, couscous cooks up light and fluffy in just a few minutes.

Cracked Wheat

Cracked wheat is made by cracking the whole wheat kernel between rollers. It is not precooked. Cracked wheat cooks very quickly and can be used as a breakfast cereal or a side dish.

Farina

Whole wheat farina is similar to cracked wheat, only finer. It makes a hearty breakfast cereal. Most farina is made from refined wheat, which does not contain the germ or bran. We recommend that you use only whole grain farina.

Rolled Wheat

Rolled wheat is the whole wheat kernel that has been steamed and then rolled between rollers to produce large thick flakes. Rolled wheat looks similar to rolled oats and can be used as a substitute for oatmeal.

Wheat Berries

Wheat berries or wheat groats are the whole grain kernels of hard red wheat. When cooked, they are chewy and substantial. They can be used in pilafs and as the basis of a casserole. To minimize cooking time, wheat berries should be soaked overnight or for 4 to 6 hours in water before cooking.

Wheat Germ

Wheat germ is the germ or embryo of the wheat seed. It is rich in oils and protein and is an excellent source of the B vitamins. Because of its oil content, wheat germ should always be refrigerated to prevent it from becoming rancid. Wheat germ can be sprinkled on hot cereal and added to other grain dishes to increase their nutrient content.

Wheat Bran

Wheat bran is the outer coat of the wheat kernel. It is one of the best sources of insoluble fiber. Wheat bran can be sprinkled on hot cereals or added to other grain dishes.

How to Use Wheat

There is a form of wheat for each meal of the day. Rolled wheat and farina make excellent breakfast cereals. Wheat berries can be substitute for rice and used in stuffings and pilafs. Bulgur, cracked wheat, and couscous make wonderful side dishes.

Store whole grains in airtight containers out of direct sunlight. They will keep for about six to nine months. Wheat germ should be stored in the refrigerator for up to three months or in your freezer for six to nine months.

Recipes

Basic Cooking Instructions

To presoak: Add berries and cooking liquid to rice bowl and let sit overnight or during the day in refrigerator.

1 cup wheat berries
1 cup water, juice, or broth
Salt to taste

Plastic Steamers
Fill reservoir to maximum with water and turn on machine. Steam for 50 to 60 minutes. Season and serve.

Metal Steamers
Coat rice bowl with nonstick spray. Add grain and water to rice bowl with an additional 1½ cups of water and turn on machine. After machine turns off, let steam for 5 minutes on warm. Season and serve.

Serves 4

Nutrition Facts

Serving Size 1.693 ounces (48.00g)
Servings Per Container 1

Amount Per Serving

Calories 157   Calories from Fat 7

	% *Daily Value**
Total Fat 1g	2%
Saturated Fat 0g	0%
Cholesterol 0mg	0%
Sodium 1mg	0%
Total Carbohydrate 34g	11%
Dietary Fiber 3g	12%
Sugars 0g	
Protein 6g	

Vitamin A 0%	Vitamin C 0%
Calcium 1%	Iron 8%

---

*Percent Daily Values are based on a 2,000 calorie diet. Your daily values may be higher or lower depending on your calorie needs.

Indian Breakfast Uppuma

This South Indian dish is a hearty winter warm-up meal.

½ teaspoon black mustard seeds
1 medium onion, chopped
½ green pepper, chopped
1 tablespoon oil
2 cups water
1 cup cracked wheat
Juice of ½ lemon
⅛ teaspoon turmeric powder
Salt to taste
½ tablespoon finely grated fresh ginger root (optional)
¼ cup cashew pieces (optional)
¼ cup raisins (optional)

Plastic Steamers

Fill reservoir to maximum with water and turn on machine. Sauté mustard seeds, onion, and green pepper in oil. When onion is translucent, add this mixture to grain steamer along with water and cracked wheat. Steam for 15 to 20 minutes. Season and serve.

Metal Steamers

Coat rice bowl with nonstick spray. Sauté mustard seeds, onion, and green pepper in oil. When onion is translucent, add this mixture to grain steamer along with water plus an additional ¼ cup and cracked wheat. After machine turns off, season and let steam for 1 or 2 minutes on warm.

Serves 4

Nutrition Facts

Serving Size 3.434 ounces (97.35g)
Servings Per Container 4

Amount Per Serving

Calories 203   Calories from Fat 40

	% Daily Value*
Total Fat 4g	6%
Saturated Fat 1g	5%
Cholesterol 0mg	0%
Sodium 3mg	0%
Total Carbohydrate 37g	12%
Dietary Fiber 3g	12%
Sugars 1g	
Protein 7g	

Vitamin A 0%	Vitamin C 32%
Calcium 2%	Iron 10%

*Percent Daily Values are based on a 2,000 calorie diet. Your daily values may be higher or lower depending on your calorie needs.

Bulgur Pilaf with Mushrooms

This dish reheats well, so make a batch on the weekend and you'll have dinner taken care of for the following days.

2 cups water
2 cups bulgur
2 cups sliced, fresh mushrooms
1 medium onion
⅓ cup toasted pumpkin seeds
¼ cup currants
1 tablespoon sesame oil
Shoyu or tamari to taste

Plastic Steamers
Fill reservoir to maximum with water and turn on machine. Steam for 15 to 20 minutes. Season and serve.

Metal Steamers
Coat rice bowl with nonstick spray. Add ingredients to rice bowl plus an additional ½ cup of water and turn on machine. After machine turns off, season and let steam for 1 or 2 minutes on warm. Season and let grain steam for 5 minutes before serving.

Serves 8

Nutrition Facts	
Serving Size 2.481 ounces (70.34g)	
Servings Per Container 8	
Amount Per Serving	
Calories 157 Calories from Fat 25	
	% *Daily Value**
Total Fat 3g	5%
Saturated Fat 0g	0%
Cholesterol 0mg	0%
Sodium 7mg	0%
Total Carbohydrate 30g	10%
Dietary Fiber 10g	40%
Sugars 1g	
Protein 5g	
Vitamin A 0%	Vitamin C 4%
Calcium 1%	Iron 6%

*Percent Daily Values are based on a 2,000 calorie diet. Your daily values may be higher or lower depending on your calorie needs.

Apple Cinnamon Couscous

The couscous really picks up the flavor of the apple juice. Children love this sweet treat.

1 cup apple juice
1 cup couscous
1 red delicious apple
1 teaspoon cinnamon
Salt to taste

Plastic Steamers
Fill reservoir to maximum with water, add ingredients and turn on machine. Steam for 15 to 20 minutes. Season and serve.

Metal Steamers
Coat rice bowl with nonstick spray. Add ingredients to rice bowl with an additional ¼ cup water and turn on machine. After machine turns off, season and let steam for 1 or 2 minutes on warm.

Serves 4

Nutrition Facts	
Serving Size 7.287 ounces (206.6g)	
Servings Per Container 4	
Amount Per Serving	
Calories 254 Calories from Fat 5	
	% *Daily Value**
Total Fat 1g	2%
Saturated Fat 0g	0%
Cholesterol 0mg	0%
Sodium 9mg	0%
Total Carbohydrate 56g	19%
Dietary Fiber 8g	32%
Sugars 5g	
Protein 6g	
Vitamin A 0%	Vitamin C 89%
Calcium 2%	Iron 6%

*Percent Daily Values are based on a 2,000 calorie diet. Your daily values may be higher or lower depending on your calorie needs.

Bulgur with Fresh Corn and Pumpkin Seeds

The sweet corn, salty miso, bitter parsley, and sour lemon give this recipe the full range of flavors that make it so rich.

1 cup bulgur wheat
1½ cups water
⅛ cup miso paste
½ tablespoon tamari or soy sauce
½ cup frozen or fresh corn kernals
⅛ cup pumpkin seeds, toasted
⅛ cup parsley or green onions, thinly sliced for garnish
½ tablespoon lemon juice

Plastic Steamers
Fill reservoir to minimum with water and turn on machine. Mix bulgur, water, miso, soy sauce, corn, and seeds in steamer bowl or pan and cook for 15 to 20 minutes. When bulgur is tender, remove from pan to a serving dish and garnish with parsley or green onions. Season and serve.

Metal Steamers
Coat rice bowl with nonstick spray. Mix bulgur, water, miso, soy sauce, corn, seeds, and an additional ¼ cup water in steamer bowl and steam. After machine turns off, let steam for 5 minutes before serving. Remove from pan to a serving dish and garnish with parsley or green onions.

Serves 4

Nutrition Facts	
Serving Size 2.977 ounces (84.41g)	
Servings Per Container 4	
Amount Per Serving	
Calories 221 Calories from Fat 32	
	% *Daily Value**
Total Fat 4g	6%
Saturated Fat 1g	5%
Cholesterol 0mg	0%
Sodium 445mg	19%
Total Carbohydrate 43g	14%
Dietary Fiber 4g	16%
Sugars 1g	
Protein 9g	
Vitamin A 1%	Vitamin C 5%
Calcium 2%	Iron 15%

*Percent Daily Values are based on a 2,000 calorie diet. Your daily values may be higher or lower depending on your calorie needs.

Cracked Wheat Porridge

Children will love this creamy and sweet cereal.

1 cup water
⅔ cup cracked wheat
⅓ cup creamy wheat farina
1 cup dried apple slices, chopped
1 teaspoon cinnamon powder
1 teaspoon vanilla extract

Optional: Add up to ¼ cup of any combination of the following: slivered almonds, raisins, sesame or sunflower seeds. Finely chopped fresh apple pieces can be used in place of the dried apple slices.

Serve with milk and honey as you would a traditional porridge.

Plastic Steamers
Fill reservoir to maximum with water and turn on machine. Add ingredients and steam for 15 to 20 minutes. Season and serve.

Metal Steamers
Coat rice bowl with nonstick spray. Add ingredients to rice bowl with an additional ¼ cup water and turn on machine. After machine turns off, season and let steam for 1 or 2 minutes on warm.

Serves 4

Nutrition Facts	
Serving Size 4.879 ounces (138.3g)	
Servings Per Container 4	
Amount Per Serving	
Calories 125 Calories from Fat 6	
	% *Daily Value**
Total Fat 1g	2%
Saturated Fat 0g	0%
Cholesterol 0mg	0%
Sodium 21mg	1%
Total Carbohydrate 29g	10%
Dietary Fiber 2g	8%
Sugars 0g	
Protein 3g	
Vitamin A 0%	Vitamin C 0%
Calcium 1%	Iron 6%

*Percent Daily Values are based on a 2,000 calorie diet. Your daily values may be higher or lower depending on your calorie needs.

Wheat Berry Salad

A lowfat protein-rich salad. This dressing works well on a variety of grains.

2 cups cooked, cooled wheat berries
½ cup halved seedless grapes

Green Dressing

1 cup lowfat cottage cheese
2 tablespoons torn fresh basil leaves
1 tablespoon fresh lemon juice
Salt to taste

To make dressing, combine ingredients in a blender or food processor until smooth. Toss berries and grapes with dressing.

Serves 4

Nutrition Facts

Serving Size 3.178 ounces (90.11g)
Servings Per Container 4

Amount Per Serving

Calories 192   Calories from Fat 12

	% Daily Value*
Total Fat 1g	2%
Saturated Fat 0g	0%
Cholesterol 2mg	1%
Sodium 116mg	5%
Total Carbohydrate 38g	13%
Dietary Fiber 3g	12%
Sugars 3g	
Protein 10g	

Vitamin A 0%	Vitamin C 2%
Calcium 3%	Iron 10%

*Percent Daily Values are based on a 2,000 calorie diet. Your daily values may be higher or lower depending on your calorie needs.

CHAPTER 19

Wild Rice (Zizania aquatica)

This aquatic grass seed is dark brown and twiglike and has a distinctive woodsy flavor and pleasant, chewy texture.

Wild rice is native to the Great Lakes region of the Midwest and for years was hand-cultivated by the Chippewa. It is the seed of a wild aquatic grass that grows in the shallow moving waters at the inlets and outlets of lakes in central North America, particularly in the lake regions of western Ontario, eastern Manitoba, Wisconsin, and Minnesota. In these regions, wild rice was once the staple food of the Native Americans.

What Is Wild Rice?

Wild rice is not a rice and not a real grain. It is the seed from a plume-topped, wild aquatic plant that is native to North America. The dark brown grains are longer and thinner than real rice and turn slightly purple when cooked. Wild rice is expensive due to short supply and hand gathering and thrashing.

Nutrition and Wild Rice

Wild rice is an excellent source of protein as well as the B vitamins thiamin, riboflavin, niacin, folate, and pyridoxine. It is also a good source of the minerals magnesium, zinc, iron, and copper. The bran of wild rice is rich in insoluble fiber.

How to Buy Wild Rice

Wild rice is usually sold in boxes or as part of a mixture of grains. Wild rice can be purchased in bulk bins at some health food or specialty stores.

Wild Rice

Wild rice can be found in supermarkets, gourmet food stores, and health food stores. If you cannot locate it, contact one of the mail order companies in the back of the book.

Wild Rice and Brown Rice Mix

Wild rice is expensive. Often it is mixed with brown rice to make pilaf mixes. Look for these mixes in supermarkets, specialty stores, health food stores, or the mail order companies listed in the back of the book. When choosing a mix, look for one that does not contain MSG, artificial colors, flavors, or modified starch.

How to Use Wild Rice

Wild rice can be used in poultry dressings, salads, soups, casseroles, and in any recipe that calls for rice. Try mixing wild rice with other grains. Wild rice especially complements the taste and texture of brown rice.

Wild rice should be put in a sealed container and stored in a cool, dark place.

Recipes

Basic Cooking Instructions

Wild rice is extremely hard. The cooking time can be greatly reduced by presoaking.

Many people consider wild rice overcooked if the grains burst open. However, we like this grain cooked to the point where the grains open and curl. Not only are they soft and easily chewed this way, the variety of colors and shapes makes them very eye-appealing.

1 cup wild rice
1 cup water, juice, or broth
Salt to taste

To presoak: Add wild rice and cooking liquid to rice bowl and let sit overnight or 6 to 8 hours during the day in refrigerator.

Plastic Steamers

Fill reservoir to maximum with water and turn on machine. Steam for 50 to 60 minutes. Season and serve.

Metal Steamers

Coat rice bowl with nonstick spray. Add ingredients to rice bowl plus an additional 1½ cups water and turn on machine. After machine turns off, season and let steam for 1 or 2 minutes on warm.

Serves 4

Nutrition Facts	
Serving Size 1.411 ounces (40.00g)	
Servings Per Container 4	
Amount Per Serving	
Calories 143 Calories from Fat 4	
	% *Daily Value**
Total Fat 0g	0%
Saturated Fat 0g	0%
Cholesterol 0mg	0%
Sodium 3mg	0%
Total Carbohydrate 30g	10%
Dietary Fiber 1g	4%
Sugars 0g	
Protein 6g	
Vitamin A 0%	Vitamin C 0%
Calcium 0%	Iron 4%

*Percent Daily Values are based on a 2,000 calorie diet. Your daily values may be higher or lower depending on your calorie needs.

Wild Breakfast Rice

Live dangerously and start the day on the wild side with this unusual cereal.

1 cup water
½ cup wild rice, presoaked
½ cup short-grain brown rice
2 tablespoons molasses
Salt to taste
¼ cup finely chopped dried sour cherries
¼ cup date sugar

Plastic Steamers

Fill reservoir to maximum with water and turn on machine. Add water, wild rice, brown rice, molasses, and salt and steam for 50 to 60 minutes. Add cherries during last 30 minutes of steaming time. Top cereal with date sugar.

Metal Steamers

Coat rice bowl with nonstick spray. Add water, wild rice, brown rice, and an additional 1½ cups of water to rice bowl and turn on machine. After machine turns off, stir in molasses and salt and let steam for 1 or 2 minutes on warm. Top cereal with date sugar.

Serves 4

Nutrition Facts	
Serving Size 2.538 ounces (71.96g)	
Servings Per Container 4	
Amount Per Serving	
Calories 235 Calories from Fat 9	
	% *Daily Value**
Total Fat 1g	2%
Saturated Fat 0g	0%
Cholesterol 0mg	0%
Sodium 13mg	1%
Total Carbohydrate 53g	18%
Dietary Fiber 2g	8%
Sugars 11g	
Protein 5g	
Vitamin A 6%	Vitamin C 8%
Calcium 9%	Iron 15%

*Percent Daily Values are based on a 2,000 calorie diet. Your daily values may be higher or lower depending on your calorie needs.

Wild Rice Salad with Apples and Walnuts

A wonderful change of pace from rice salads. We like our wild rice "overcooked" so that the grains burst and curl.

2 cups cooked wild rice
1 cup coarsely chopped walnuts
1 cup raisins
1 medium red apple (not delicious), cored and diced
1 celery rib, sliced
4 scallions, thinly sliced
1 tablespoon vegetable oil
¼ teaspoon salt
Grated rind of 1 lemon

Dressing

2 tablespoons lemon juice
2 tablespoons olive oil
2 tablespoons finely chopped cilantro
1 garlic clove

To make dressing, combine ingredients in blender and process until smooth.

Toss salad ingredients together and pour dressing over them. Let sit for 1 hour. Serve on a bed of lettuce if desired.

Serves 6

Nutrition Facts	
Serving Size 5.4 ounces (152.1g)	
Servings Per Container 6	
Amount Per Serving	
Calories 322 Calories from Fat 151	
	% *Daily Value**
Total Fat 17g	26%
Saturated Fat 1g	5%
Cholesterol 0mg	0%
Sodium 21mg	1%
Total Carbohydrate 40g	13%
Dietary Fiber 4g	16%
Sugars 4g	
Protein 8g	
Vitamin A 3%	Vitamin C 15%
Calcium 3%	Iron 10%

*Percent Daily Values are based on a 2,000 calorie diet. Your daily values may be higher or lower depending on your calorie needs.

Wild Rice and Cranberries

We like this because it's simple, delicious, and looks great. It can be served hot or cold.

1 cup wild rice, cooked with lowfat chicken broth
1 cup dried cranberries
½ cup raisins
Salt to taste

Combine ingredients and serve.

Serves 4

Nutrition Facts	
Serving Size 3.862 ounces (109.5g)	
Servings Per Container 4	
Amount Per Serving	
Calories 96 Calories from Fat 3	
	% *Daily Value**
Total Fat 0g	0%
Saturated Fat 0g	0%
Cholesterol 0mg	0%
Sodium 3mg	0%
Total Carbohydrate 21g	7%
Dietary Fiber 2g	8%
Sugars 1g	
Protein 3g	
Vitamin A 0% Vitamin C 6%	
Calcium 0% Iron 3%	

*Percent Daily Values are based on a 2,000 calorie diet. Your daily values may be higher or lower depending on your calorie needs.

Wild Rice Pilaf

This Eastern dish gets a Southwest twist with the help of a little cumin.

½ cup cooked wild rice (made with chicken broth)
½ cup cooked long-grain brown rice (made with chicken broth)
1 clove garlic, minced
½ teaspoon cumin
Cilantro (optional)

Mix all ingredients and serve warm or cold. Garnish with cilantro if desired.

Serves 4

Nutrition Facts	
Serving Size 3.718 ounces (105.4g)	
Servings Per Container 4	

Amount Per Serving

Calories 170	Calories from Fat 12
	% Daily Value*
Total Fat 1g	2%
Saturated Fat 0g	0%
Cholesterol 0mg	0%
Sodium 198mg	8%
Total Carbohydrate 34g	11%
Dietary Fiber 2g	8%
Sugars 0g	
Protein 6g	

Vitamin A 0%	Vitamin C 0%
Calcium 1%	Iron 6%

*Percent Daily Values are based on a 2,000 calorie diet. Your daily values may be higher or lower depending on your calorie needs.

Mail Order Companies

Arrowhead Mills
110 South Lawton
Hereford, TX 79045
(806) 364-0730

Bob's Red Mill
Natural Foods, Inc.
5209 S.E. International Way
Milwaukee, Oregon 97222
(503) 654-3215
This company sells whole grains including ancient grains such as teff, quinoa, and spelt. They also have an extensive catalog boasting such quality products as whole amaranth, pearl barley, and buckwheat groats. They carry many of the hard-to-find products and have an outstanding customer service department.

Deer Valley Farm
P.O. Box 173
Guilford, NY 13780-0173
(607) 764-8556
Call for a free catalog. This company carries grains and seeds such as kamut, spelt, and quinoa.

Niblack Foods, Inc.
900 Jefferson Road, Bldg. #5
Rochester, NY 14623
(716) 292-0790
1-800-724-8883

Send for a price list. This company carries many whole grain baking products as well as whole grains such as quinoa, amaranth, spelt, and kamut. They supply commercial bakers and can handle orders of large quantities.

Sam Wylde
P.O. Box 84488
Seattle, WA 98124
(206) 762-5400
1-800-325-9788

Call for a free catalog. This is the parent company for Ener-G Foods (manufacturers of high quality whole grain baking products). They carry grain products such as wheat berries, cracked rye, cornmeal, and millet.

Walnut Acres
Penns Creek, PA 17862
1-800-433-3998

Call for a free catalog and ask for the "No-room-in-the-catalogue-sheet" that lists many of the more unusual whole grains that have been special customer requests. These include millet, spelt, quinoa, and amaranth seed. They have an impressive product list of baking goods, and packaged health foods such as nut butters, dried fruits, and soups.

Index

International Conversion Chart

These are not *exact* equivalents; they've been slightly rounded to make measuring easier.

Cup Measurements

American	Imperial	Metric	Australian
¼ cup (2 oz)	2 fl oz	60 ml	2 tablespoons
⅓ cup (3 oz)	3 fl oz	84 ml	¼ cup
½ cup (4 oz)	4 fl oz	125 ml	⅓ cup
⅔ cup (5 oz)	5 fl oz	170 ml	½ cup
¾ cup (6 oz)	6 fl oz	185 ml	⅔ cup
1 cup (8 oz)	8 fl oz	250 ml	¾ cup

Spoon Measurements

American	Metric
¼ teaspoon	1 ml
½ teaspoon	2 ml
1 teaspoon	5 ml
1 tablespoon	15 ml

Oven Temperatures

Fahrenheit	Celsius
250	120
300	150
325	160
350	180
375	190
400	200
450	230